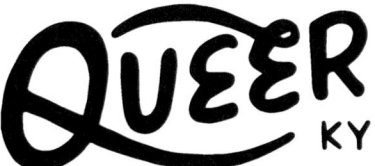

Queer Kentucky is a diverse LGBTQ+ run non-profit based in Kentucky working to bolster and enhance Queer culture and health through storytelling, education, and action. Through our storytelling approach, we give visibility and celebrate the lives of LGBTQ+ people in the great Bluegrass State. Visibility alone is life-saving. Queer Kentucky actively works with organizations and businesses on their inclusivity efforts that enhance the well-being of their employees.

Dedication
To every Queer person struggling, and to all those who have succumbed to their struggles.
Please know you aren't alone.

And to the thriving LGBTQ+ people and allies working to enhance the lives of our community.

We see you fighting, and we're standing with you.

DONATE/SUBSCRIBE

Copyright © 2025 by Queer Kentucky
All rights reserved.
Queer Kentucky
PO Box 424
Covington, KY 41012

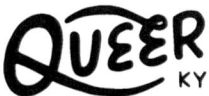

Executive Director
Missy Spears

Editor-in-Chief
Spencer Jenkins

Design
Brackish Creative

Contributing photographers and artists
Alexey Kim aka Sidewalkkilla
Carey Neal Gough
Faulkner Morgan Archive
Jeremy Grier
Jon Cherry
Kaybee Photo
Logan Oleson
Ryan Grant
Scotty Milks

Contributing writers
Basel Touchan
Belle Townsend
Bryan Hall
Duncan Cherry
Faulkner Morgan Archive
Imani N. Dennison
Sirene Martin
Spencer Adkins
Vic Leon

Web development
Honeywick

For advertising inquiries
contact@Queerkentucky.com

CONTENTS

QUEEN OUT OR GET OUT 28

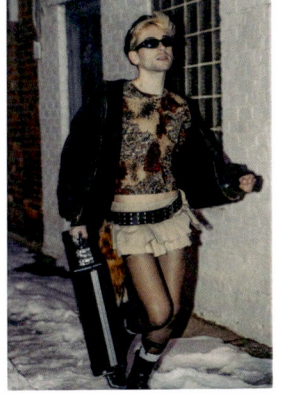

36 THE BEST GAY ONE-NIGHT STAND IN AMERICA

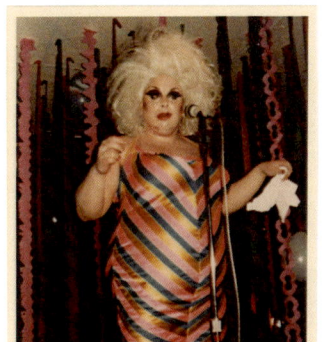

FROM NO STOPLIGHTS TO HER NAME IN LIGHTS 40

46 BOONE COUNTY TO BARTSCHLAND

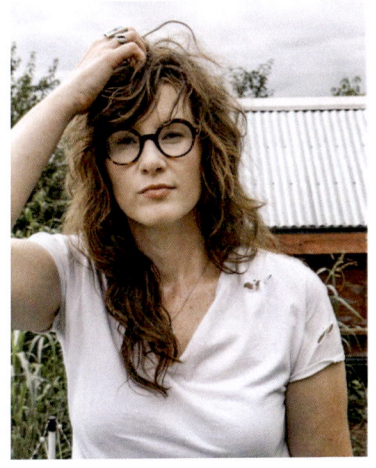

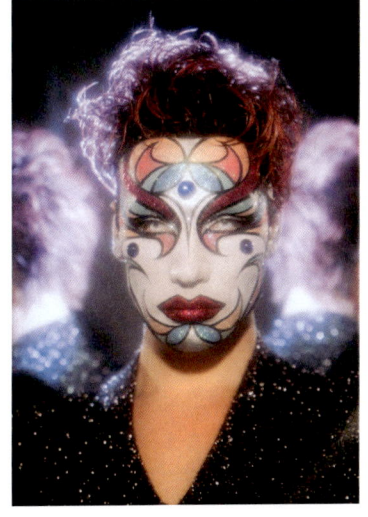

ZACK WICKHAM'S LOVE LETTER TO LOUISVILLE 62

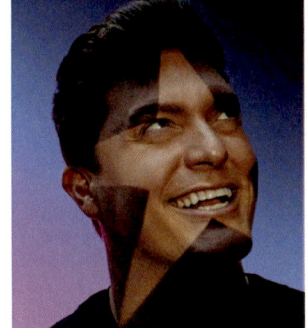

AND

06. A TOAST TO CHAMPAGNE
14. FROM SPOTLIGHT TO SHADOW AND BACK AGAIN
20. BUILDING BRIDGES FOR RURAL QUEER ARTISTS
24. PERFORMANCE AS RESISTANCE
54. PERFORMING OUR POWER
58. NEEDING NO MEETING PLACE
70. BRINGING OUT THE ELVIS

DEAR READER,

When I was a kid, I dedicated an entire summer to playing the narrator in the musical *Beauty and the Beast*. Yes, the character that you actually never see in the Disney cartoon movie version. The one that delivers lines for the first 45 seconds of the film and is never heard from again—that was me. I also shuffled around the stage as a knife alongside a posse of utensils to the number, "Be Our Guest." Needless to say, I wasn't the prime pick for any leading roles.

But that was fine with me. Who doesn't love a supporting role? Some of the most powerful performances come from those who set the stage for others. Viola Davis won an Oscar for *Doubt* with just one monologue—one monologue filled with raw emotion (and a lot of snot).

As for the leading role of the Beast, my childhood bestie was cast. Was I jealous of his newly acquired stardom? Not really, I didn't necessarily want to be there. His mom had pushed my mom to push me into this summer camp, so there I was supporting Miss Thang in her furry beast costume, while she fought off the evil Gaston and won Belle's heart.

And support I did! I donned that elementary school stage in my best 18th-Century French attire, brown from head to toe. My costume consisted of itchy, cotton tights; cunty leather boots; and a very blousey top, complete with a "provincial" vest.

Once upon a time, in a faraway land, a young Prince lived in a shining castle.

Although he had everything his heart desired, the Prince was spoiled, selfish, and unkind…

I slayed that prologue. I set the stage for one of the most famous love stories of all time. And now, years later, I find myself doing the same thing—but this time, the story is ours.

As your Editor-in-Chief of Queer Kentucky, I live in this constant supporting role of sharing our stories with readers all over the world. I get the privilege of reading, writing and editing so many Queer stories of joy. I uplift your business milestones, your inspiring advocacy wins, and beautiful works of art with digital heart taps and freshly printed paper. And the process is beautiful, even the hot-off-the-press odor of this magazine is beautiful.

But just as *Beauty and the Beast* begins with a curse before love breaks the spell, our stories of joy exist alongside struggle. Queer Kentucky's origin story is rooted in joy, but joy is impossible to fully appreciate without first knowing sorrow. That means I also have the heavy responsibility of sharing stories of hate, political violence, destruction, and even death. I don't enjoy writing about transgender trauma, "drag bans," or guns being pulled on Queer kids at an Appalachian Pride event. But these are our stories. This is part of our history—a history they are trying to erase.

And truthfully, I regret to inform you that I don't know what happens next. I wish, dear reader, that this letter would bring you joy and not root you in a reality of worry for our Queer future. But that doesn't mean we can't find joy. I look for it everywhere. And I find it. Through tight embraces with my chosen family, I find it. When they read me for filth to the point of me blushing in embarrassment, I find it. The joy I feel when I am surrounded by other Queer people living relentlessly and authentically in the face of erasure and political violence is incomparable.

The world can take a lot of things away from Queer people—our rights, our mainstream spaces, our healthcare, and who knows what else. But we are in charge of our joy. As long as we allow ourselves to find that joy in our little community corners of the world, they will never win, and our show will go on.

Performance shows up in the lives of Queer people every day. We perform through our crafts, like drag and art. Or we perform for the world as loud activists fighting back. Or we perform by code-switching while navigating fear and oppression. And we are weary of the performances of our allies…are they authentic in their support or is it simply….performance? Yet, no matter the stage or the role, the Queer experience never breaks, and the show must go on.

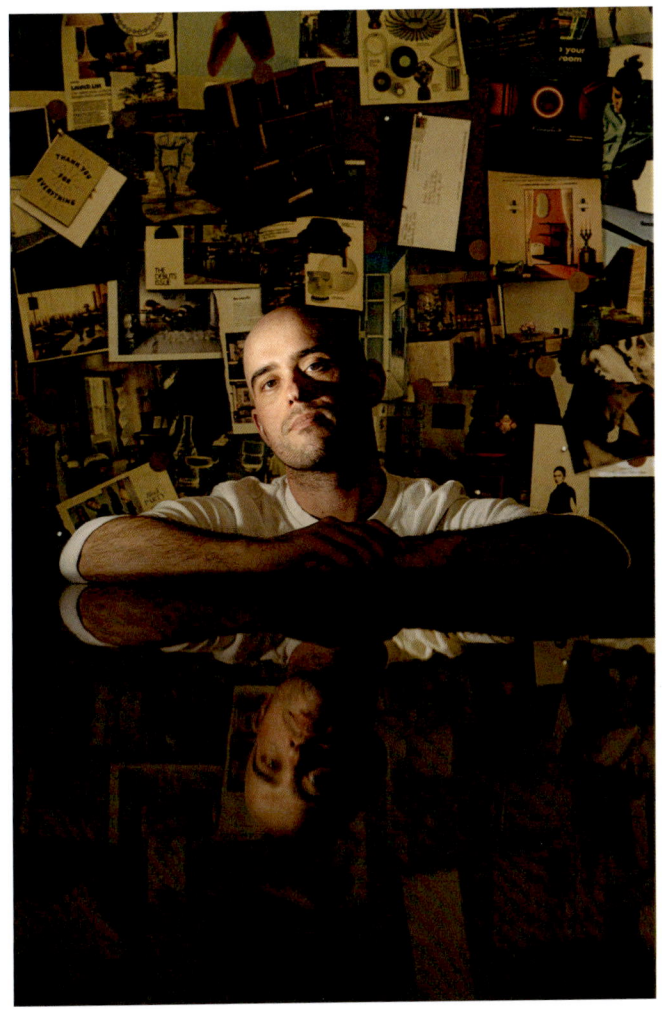

Image by Jon Cherry   he/him   @jonpcherry

I MAY HAVE KEPT THE $50K FROM TARGET.

I've been thinking a lot about the many roles I myself perform as a Queer leader. At 25, I was uncompromising in my activism. I marched, boycotted, protested—fearlessly embodying the "with us or against us" mindset. Back then, I believed any compromise was a betrayal, and I was shocked, even disgusted, when older leaders chose pragmatism over principle. I swore I'd never follow their path.

But life has a way of evolving our perspectives. At 45, I make decisions that 25-year-old me wouldn't understand—and probably wouldn't forgive. I've learned that leadership is rarely black and white. It's a balancing act where the stakes include not just yourself, but your entire community. Decisions stop being solely about what feels right to you, and start being about how the fallout of your choices trickles down. Every decision must ask, "Who gets left behind if I say no?" and "Who gets left behind if I say yes?"

Someone recently asked me why I kept a donation from a corporation that walked away from Diversity, Equity, and Inclusion. My answer wasn't simple, but my reasoning was clear. That money was promised for Queer hands, and in a community that's perpetually underfunded and underserved, rejecting those funds would have hurt far more people than it helped. Last year, over 80% of Queer Kentucky's revenue went directly into LGBTQ+ hands—over 100 writers, artists, performers, designers, influencers, journalists and more across Kentucky, Ohio, Indiana, and beyond. That's real impact. Turning away money that feeds, supports, and uplifts my community isn't a decision I get to make lightly.

Yet I wrestle with these compromises every day. Whether I'm putting on my "capitalism" hat to keep the lights on, or switching to advocacy mode in conversations about systemic change, the countless roles I perform weigh heavily. They're not all flattering, and they don't all reflect the parts of me I'm most proud of. But they make certain that the organization thrives, that the resources keep flowing, and that our Queer community continues to grow stronger.

Performance, in all its forms, is an inherent part of what it means to live and lead in the LGBTQ+ space. Sometimes, it's glorious. Sometimes, it's painful. And much of the time, it's wearing a mask, fighting in the grey area, while striving for a better world underneath it. But no matter how weary we grow, this community continuously proves its resilience.

The show must go on. And because of all of you, it will.

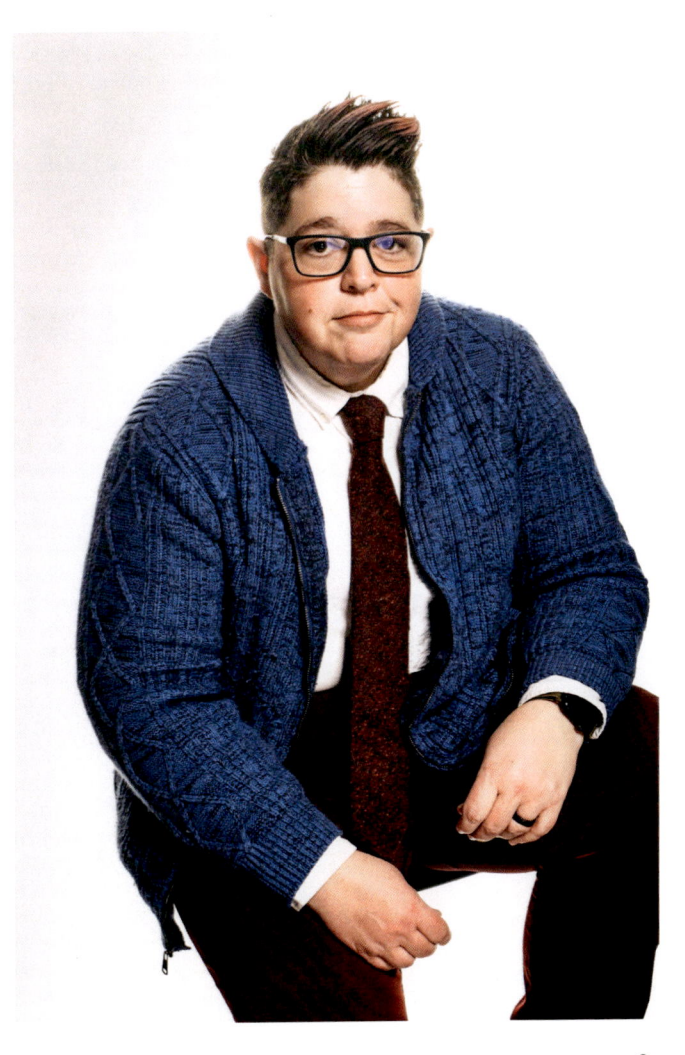

Image by Ryan Grant   he/him   @ryngrant

THE SHOW MUST GO ON

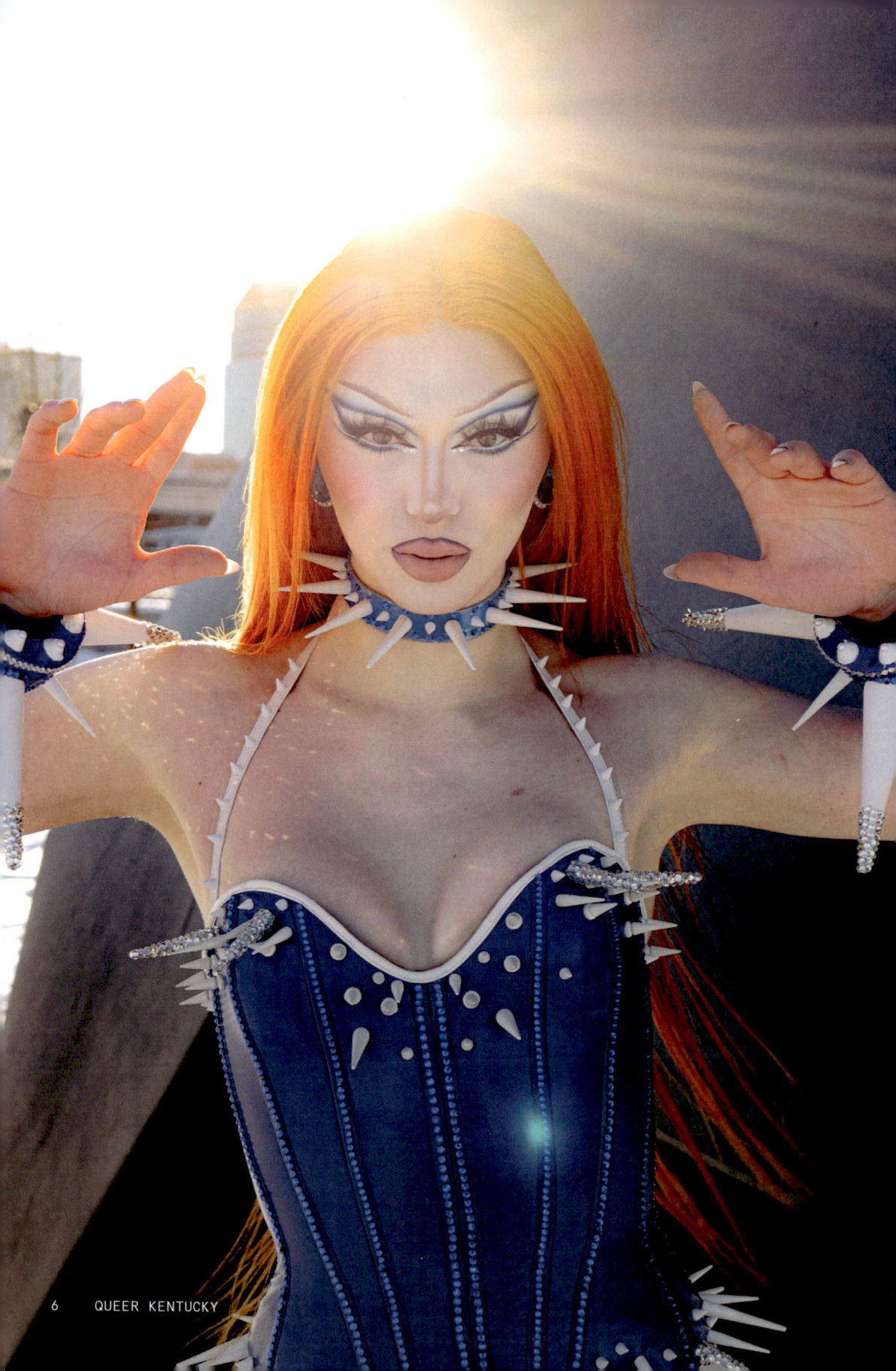

A TOAST TO CHAMPAGNE

FINDING POWER THROUGH DANCE, COMMUNITY, AND SOBRIETY

Duncan Cherry he/him   @djspringbreak

I've been attending drag shows since the first time someone sponsored me at The Connection. That may date me a bit, but also shows my long-standing appreciation for performers in this city. From the moment I saw Champagne walk on stage at PLAY Louisville, probably the same age as I was when I was invited to my first drag show, I recognized her star power. She commanded attention with effortless dancing, a perfect mug, and her captivating looks.

I first saw her perform in 2018 at Jade Jolie's Drag Me to Hell competition. She had just graduated high school and was on stage three months later. In her words, "Kind of iconic, honestly." She met her future drag mother, Uhstel H. Valentine, before she even knew what drag was. "She was just this tall goddess; you could see her across the crowd at Pride. I got a picture with her in my little homemade tie-dye pride shirt," she laughs.

Her introduction to drag, like many others, came from *RuPaul's Drag Race*. "Sophomore year I wanted to be a makeup artist," she tells me, as she glues rhinestones onto black lace fabric in her kitchen. "I saw season four of *Drag Race* and was like - 'oh my god - this is the coolest thing ever.'" We laugh, as she states that she didn't want to be a drag queen, only a makeup artist. "Being young I thought drag meant you just wanted to be a woman ... spoiler alert."

For her first performance, she spent two weeks choreographing a routine to "It's Not Right, But It's Okay" (the Thunderpuss Remix, for the girls who know) because she saw Sasha Velour perform it. "It's always that dance background," she says. Her dancing roots go back to seventh grade when she was living in Pekin, Indiana. "I moved schools and they didn't have a dance team, just this rinky-dink studio somewhere in town. I'd hang out after school, and

Images by Kaybee Photo   she/they   @ itskaybeephoto

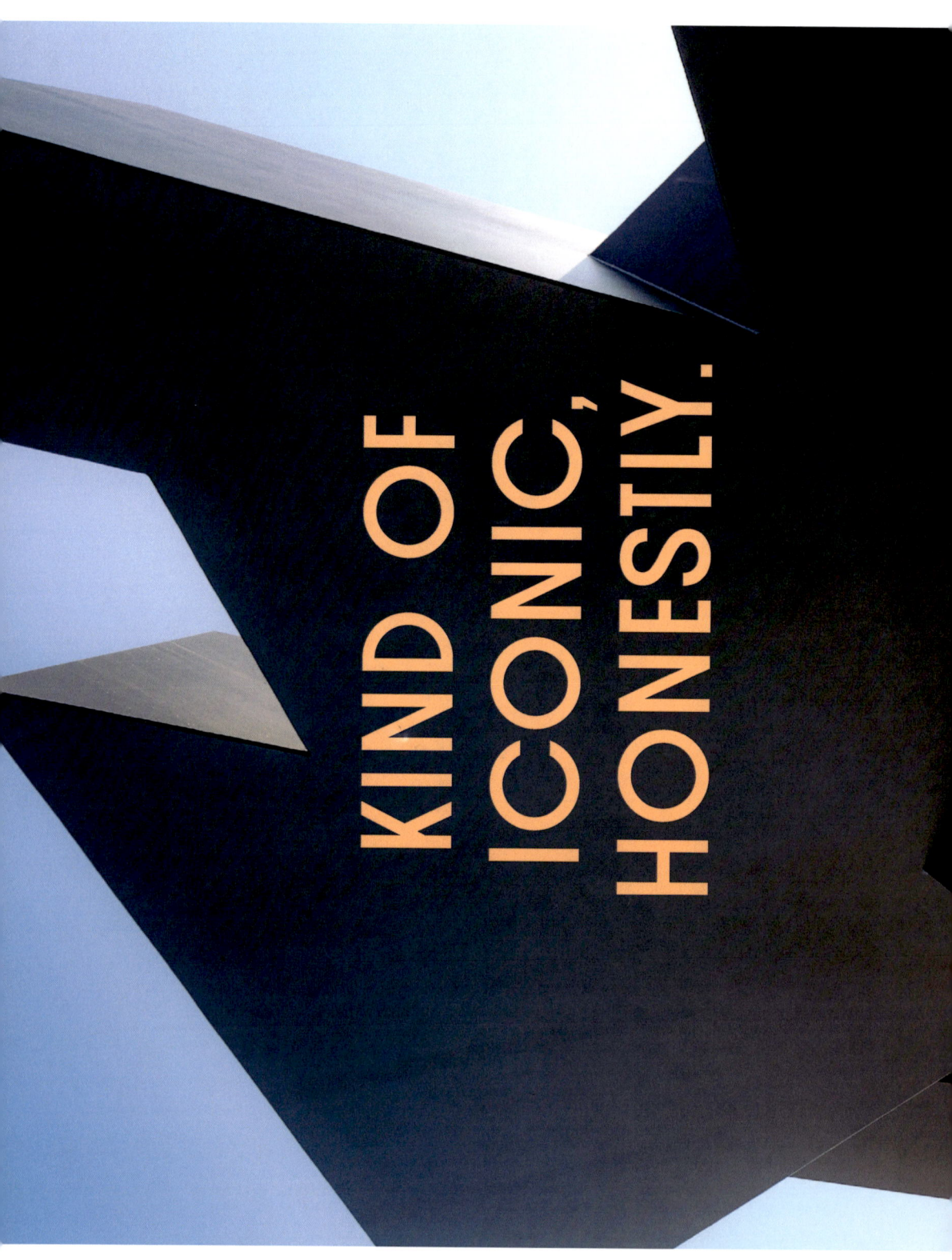

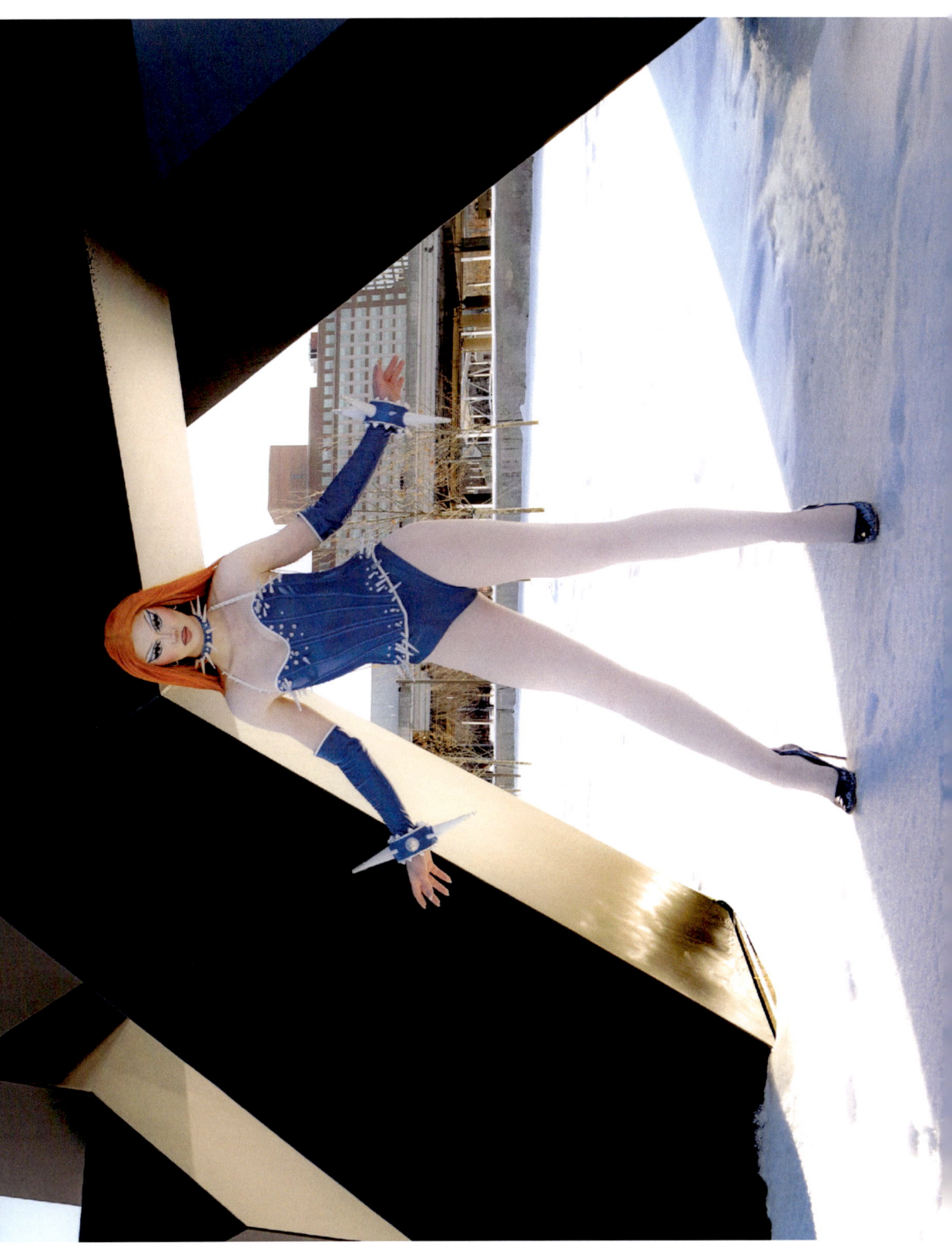

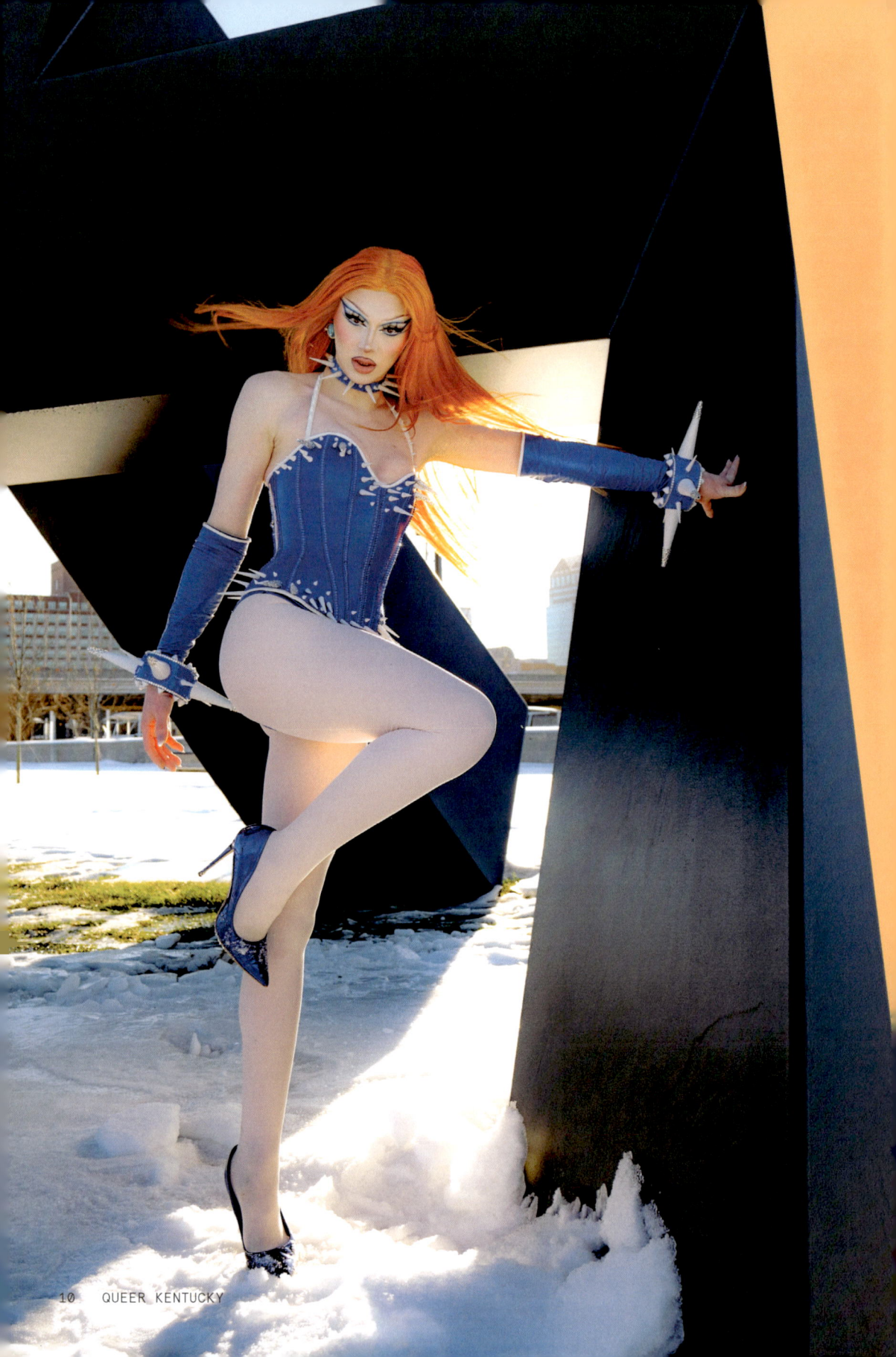

eventually got a group of people together and we started a dance team. We didn't have a real instructor - just tutorials online. We must've been pretty good because they let us perform in front of the whole school." She shrugs as she smirks proudly.

Anyone who has seen Champagne perform knows how skilled she is. Even if you haven't seen her perform, you've probably come across one of her viral videos from Drag Brunch at Le Moo, some videos reaching over six million views. She moves with grace and calculation, twirling and kicking over her head, dropping down into the splits, and perfecting any choreography from her favorite artists. "Anything Gaga," she says when I ask who she loves to channel. "She's just such a huge influence to me and I think to a lot of other Queer people. Gaga has always been a symbol of strength and self-expression for those struggling to fit in. Also I love a good Lana song — it's a slow burn, a dramatic moment in the spotlight as the main character."

As for the fine line between Champagne and Nova, her day-to-day self, she says it's less distinct than it used to be. "When I first started drag, Champagne was a character, a way to express my feminine side, and eventually [became] my trans awakening," she explains. "But now, it's hard to separate the two lives. Drag is my job, but I still feel like there's a difference when I'm 'on' compared to when I'm with my close friends. I'm bubbly and outgoing in public, but with my fiancé Nick or friends I can be more reserved."

Champagne's thoughts on the local drag scene reflect a deep awareness of the challenges the Queer community faces. "A lot of people say they support Queer art, but sometimes only online. I appreciate liking a post or sharing a video, but are they fighting for the trans and Queer community outside of that?" She pauses, her voice thoughtful. "It's stopping misinformation when you're not in your vacuum. Is it a performance online or is it who you are?"

On the topic of laws affecting Queer and trans people, she expresses concern, particularly around bathroom laws and restrictions on gender affirming care. "I haven't directly experienced it but it's worrisome, especially for young people transitioning." She feels proud that at 25, younger trans people look up to her, and that she can be someone that she didn't have in her own life during her transition. "I have people who are like, 'I just started hormones, and seeing you live your life so authentically inspires me.'" It just makes me feel good. I never thought of myself like that."

Without the luxury of as many trans elders in her life, she cites influences: "My sisters Sydni Hampton and Eris Jolie gave me good advice when I was first transitioning... advice I hope to continue with those who come after me."

We talk about her sobriety, which she's very open about. "I think it's important for people to know that everyone struggles, but there's always a path for them to grow and change," she reflects. "I don't feel like a completely new person, but I feel healthier, more compassionate, and I can focus on my journey. I'm still a bitch sometimes, but I'm a kinder one," she laughs. "Sobriety isn't a buzzkill. It opens your eyes to how you can have fun without substances. And having the solid support system of my chosen family has been key for me."

It's clear that Champagne has big plans for the future. "I want to audition for *Drag Race*, getting sober I feel like my mind is so clear on that goal." She continues, "I would love to produce my own show, a space for people to perform in a more artsy out-of-the-box way." She adds, "I'd also love to see more Queer sober spaces - places where we can hang out without needing substances. Why can't we just go bowling or have a Queer arcade?"

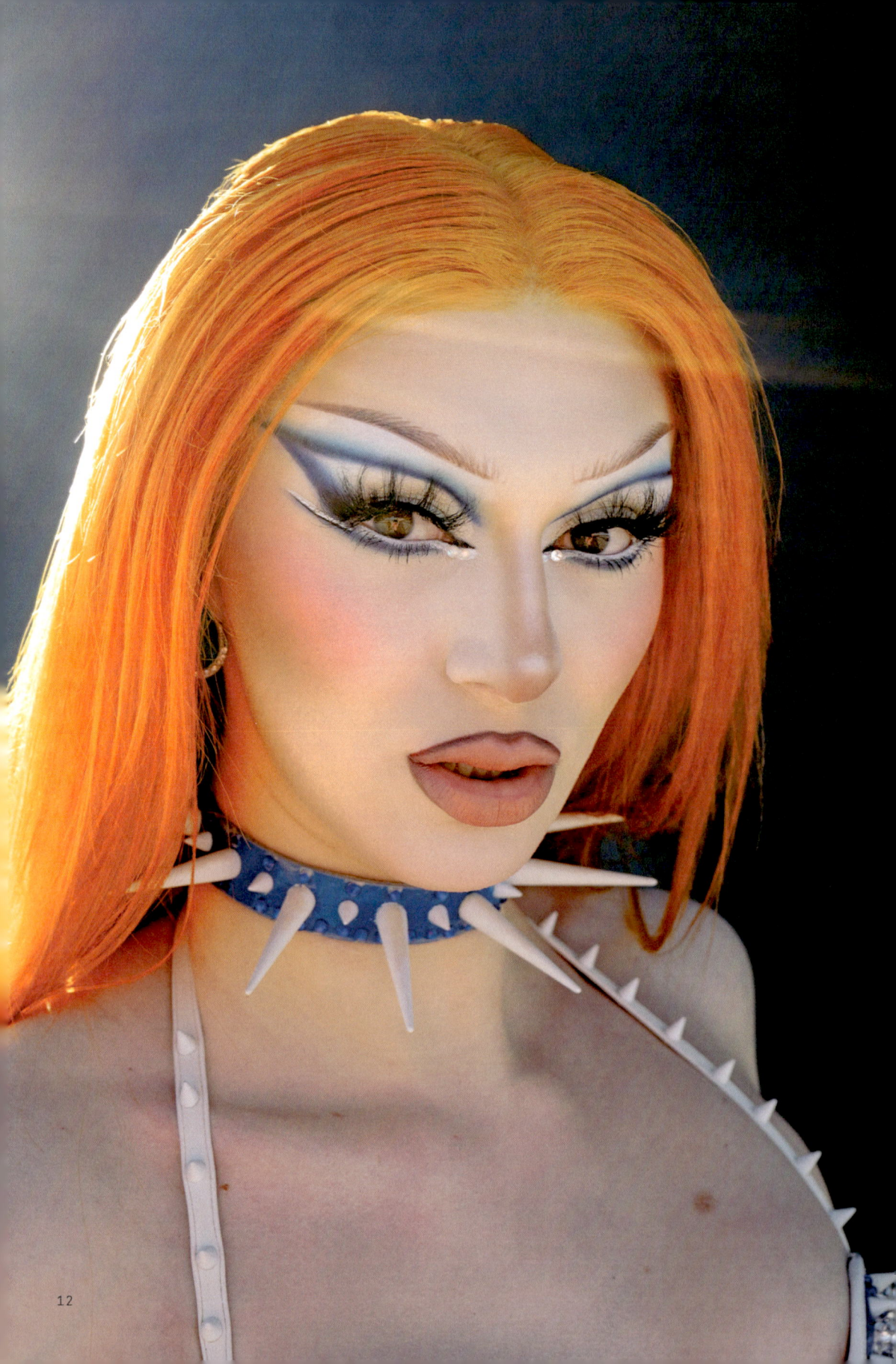

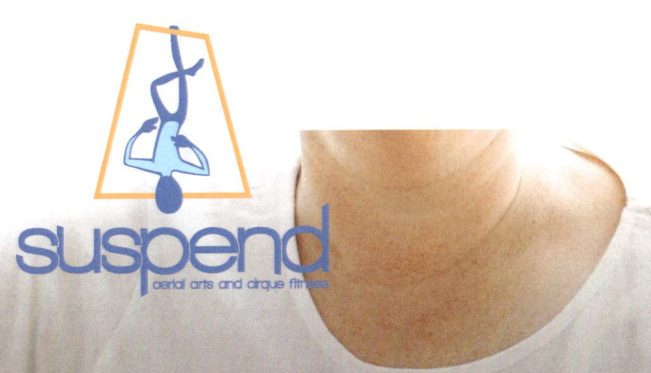

suspend
aerial arts and cirque fitness

CREATE COMMUNITY AND BECOME CENTERED AT SUSPEND LOUISVILLE.

MINDFUL MOVEMENT IS A BODY INCLUSIVE PRACTICE DESIGNED BY QUEER PEOPLE, FOR QUEER PEOPLE. FREE AND OPEN TO ALL.

SUNDAYS 10 - 10:50 A.M.
721 E WASHINGTON ST., LOUISVILLE, KY 40202

FROM SPOTLIGHT TO SHADOW AND BACK AGAIN

Bryan Hall *he/him @the.mr.bryan*

Images by Ryan Grant   he/him   @ryngrant

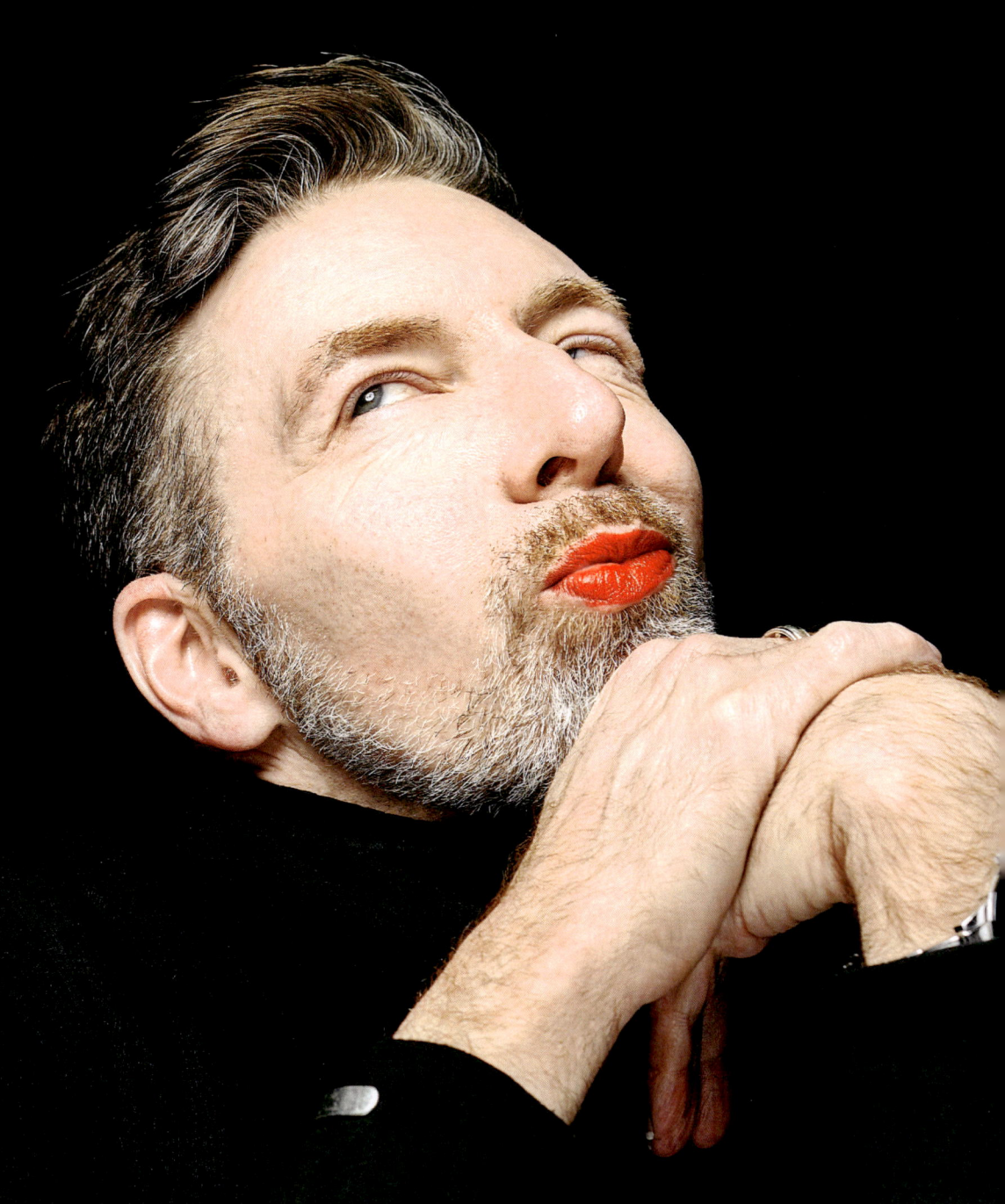

The shit-show that was life was not always so. Early in life I came to realize I was blessed with God-given talents. How did I know they were from God? Well, the talents I possessed, no one in my family possessed. No one could draw, paint, or sculpt. No one could dance, sing, or act. No one could create stories and put them to paper. So, where did these gifts that came naturally come from? My only explanation was: if it was not genetics then it must have been given by something bigger than myself; a higher power.

Of all the gifts, dance was my passion. The closest I felt to God was in the studio sweating from the execution of intricate combinations of rhythm and physical prowess. I felt the embrace of God as I turned the empty space of a stage into a canvas on which I could create visions charged with emotion, depth, and vibrancy. With dance I could be unapologetically myself. It was my therapist, my best friend, my companion, and my lover. My first true addiction.

Countless hours of literal blood, sweat, and tears made for a journey that sent me to the stars; I believed I was invincible, that nothing could get past my armor and ground me. I was sorely mistaken. I was injured during a rehearsal for the spring concert at the school I attended. Knee crushed by the misguided desires of a ballerina donning her newest dance skirt without considering her partner or the dancer's code. You never change the dancer or rehearsal code unless discussed with all who are accountable. Vanity once again preyed and fed on the defenseless, taking no prisoners. Within mere seconds I went from center stage of a prominent gilded theatre to a sterile and cold operating theatre. My career was derailed, not to mention, what I believed, my life. Makes for one hell of a resentment, coupled with a full on "back-turn" to my higher power. This is when my faith in God started to wane. This is when I turned my back on God and eventually dropped my basket.

I slowly became addicted to my painkillers, of which I slowly washed down with copious amounts of booze. Yeah, I'm that type. I couldn't have just one, in any capacity. Consistently living with the knowledge that I was a failure gnawed at my core; like the Nosferatu. Depression imprisoned me in a dark and cold cell. I was lost, and grieved over the death of the most important spiritual entity of my life. Delusion set in, and I convinced myself after a year that I had processed and healed from the event. The only thing that healed was my body. My heart, soul, and spirit were far from it. I used drugs and alcohol to mask and dull the pain of failure, the ridicule of defeat, and the utter confusion and loss of identity. When one skill set is injured another one steps in to compensate. Another talent took center stage: the actor. I could change my mask at the drop of a hat.

Though I could not soar to the rafters anymore, at least physically, I could still cut a rug. I embarked on a new journey fueled by drugs, alcohol, and denial wrapped up in makeup, rhinestones, and stilettoes. I had arrived! I was a glamorous drag queen. That's what was projected on the outside: confidence, invincibility, and grand fearlessness. On the inside I was a frightened, empty, and lonely shell of a human being.

It wasn't long before my facade started to fray and unravel, leaving me cowering at the bottom of the darkest emotional pit, devouring myself to the marrow. I single-handedly accomplished every single hedonistic, criminal, and pathetic manipulative act I swore I would never do. I betrayed my very moral fiber. I tore everything I stood for down into a pile of shit.

Looking up to the light above; I wondered, "Isn't that where I came from?" The spotlight. It came to mind that I belonged there, in the light. This would be the first step toward recovery. It happened decades ago. Yet, it took its sweet precious time to set in, so to speak. The journey has been just that: a journey. One that I wouldn't trade for the world.

I managed to claw and climb my way out, breaking my Lee press-ons and Jimmy Choo's on the way. I took the boy out of the dress and put on a new layer of costume, hiding the addiction I clung to. I became quite the functioning alcoholic. I buried my emotions and feigned well-being all the while donning a car salesman smile. My skills of manipulation blossomed so as to put a Venus flytrap to shame. This went on

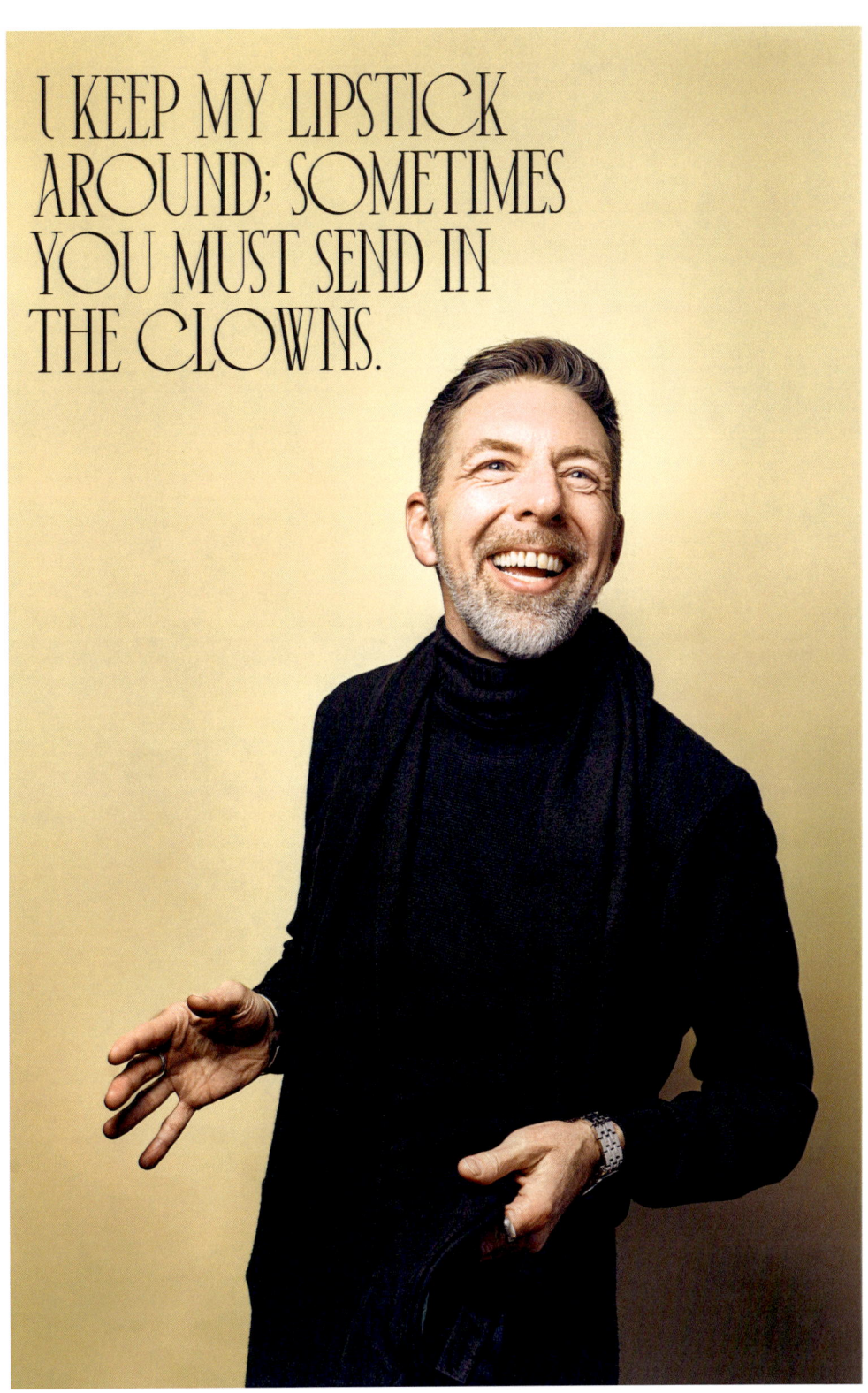

I KEEP MY LIPSTICK AROUND; SOMETIMES YOU MUST SEND IN THE CLOWNS.

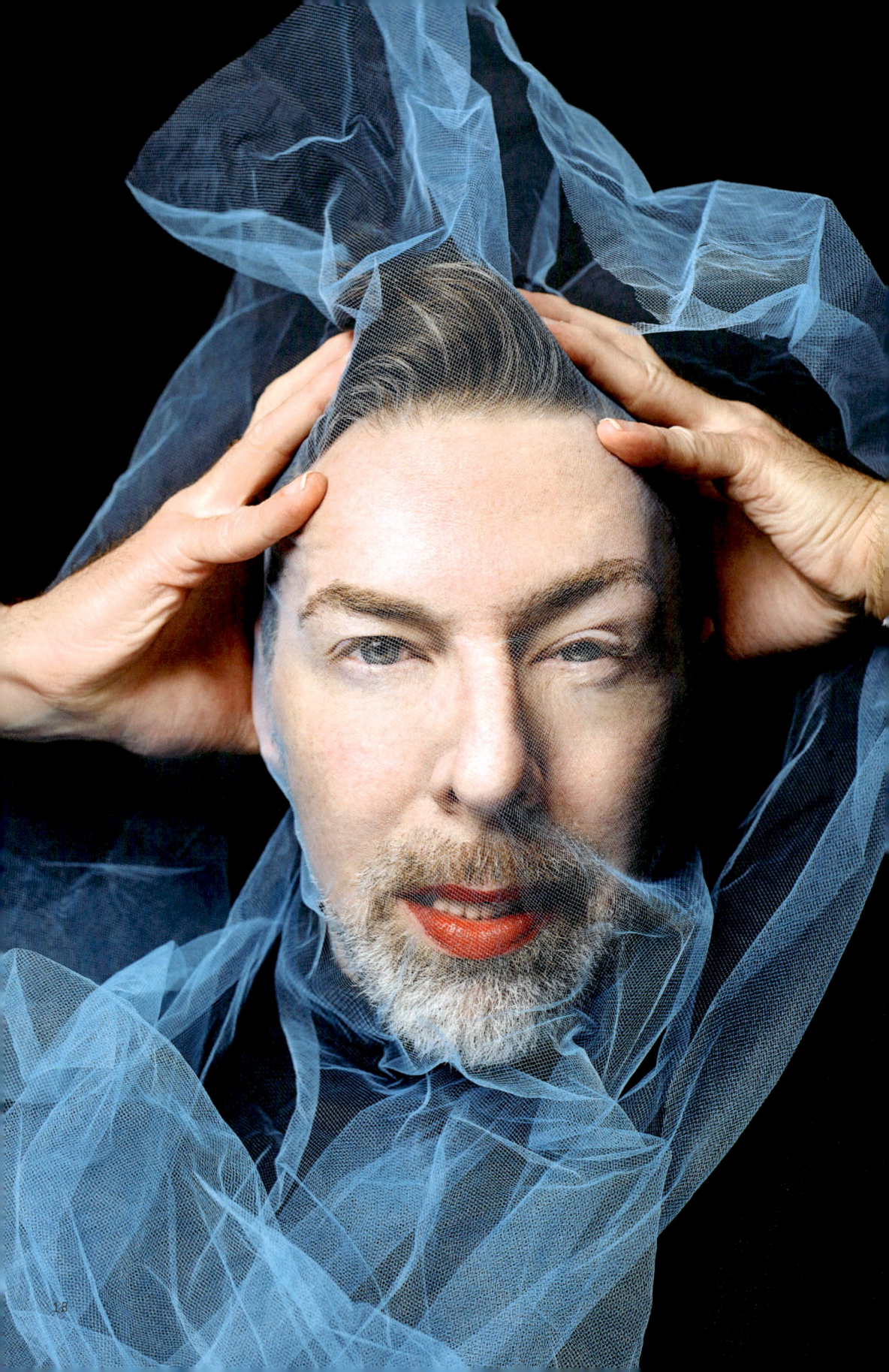

for decades through careers and relationships, each well crafted, groomed, and toxic in their own right. It was a deplorable spectacle of desperation and self-loathing.

Near the end of the show, what I thought to be the final act, I had become so isolated and despondent, so saturated with booze and self-pity that I couldn't recognize the creature in the mirror. The show had gone from a gloriously optimistic musical filled with lights and laughter to a grotesquerie filled with misery and hopelessness; the darkest of Greek tragedies. I longed for the release of it. So much so that I didn't realize I was subconsciously, systematically, and slowly committing suicide.

With the help of family, a dear friend, therapy, and what I would later come to understand was God, I finally started to wake. It was very important for me to understand that it wasn't the script that life wrote for me that was the problem. It was me. It was always me. I'm an alcoholic; I'm wired differently. Much like being a homosexual, I did not choose to be. I simply *am*. It has now been almost three years since that day. I have relapsed once in that time which lasted seven months. I wasn't finished yet. I still hadn't been convinced that I could be, much less deserved to be healthy, to love myself again. God had other plans for me. You see, even though I turned my back on God, it didn't turn it's back on me; it never left. I was always being watched over, for there are many occasions I should have not been able to get up and walk away from.

It hasn't always been easy, life still gets lifey, but it is simple if I stop trying to run the show, put in some action, gratefully play my part and follow the suggestions of a better equipped director. I keep my lipstick around; sometimes you must send in the clowns.

Thank goodness for dress rehearsals. With a new director, an ever-changing cast, and a few rewrites, the shit-show has transformed. Due to the fertilizing power of itself, it is an ever-evolving and thriving garden of love, hope, and serenity. I am eternally grateful to have a leading role in it. No matter what, life will happen, and the show must go on.

NO MATTER WHAT, LIFE WILL HAPPEN, AND THE SHOW MUST GO ON.

BUILDING BRIDGES FOR RURAL QUEER ARTISTS

MY STORY AND KENTUCKY'S CREATIVE NETWORK

Belle Townsend they/she @belletownsendky

I used to be hesitant to call myself an artist. I didn't make a living from my art, and I had no formal training. Still, my days revolved around writing whenever they could. When it felt like I had no audience, I kept writing and leaning into my art anyway. What audience did I need other than myself?

Not knowing how to navigate the traditional publishing world, I decided to self-publish my first poetry chapbook, *Push and Pull* (2022). Two more chapbooks followed: *The Observer Effect* (2023) and *The Holy in the Humdrum* (2024). Along the way, I learned that authenticity and genuine love for craft could attract an audience, even without the backing of traditional publishing.

In between these milestones, I started writing for Queer Kentucky. Through this, I discovered a vibrant and inspiring community of Queer artists across the state. The once-blurry concept of being an artist began to take shape, and the geometry wasn't as complicated as I had thought. While artistry is deeply personal, I learned that the journey doesn't have to be a solitary one.

Through Queer Kentucky and programs like New Leaders Council Kentucky and the Kentucky Rural-Urban Exchange, I uncovered the existing networks that support artists in Kentucky. After some of my videos about anti-LGBTQIA+ bills in Kentucky and poems about rural culture went viral, I found myself connected to a national community of rural and Southern people.

Leaning into this newfound community, people began reaching out for advice about opportunities for rural Queer writers. While I shared what I knew, I realized a significant gap remained, particularly for rural folks who were not straight and white. Drawing on the connections I had built across Kentucky, I decided to do something about it.

During a conversation with a peer, I mentioned my dream of creating an anthology that showcased diverse rural artists. He told me about a grant with a same-day deadline. I applied, and to my surprise, I got it. A month later, I applied for another grant and was awarded that one too.

Having never received a grant before, I felt out of my depth. The realization that being a working artist involves much more than creating—grant writing, marketing, networking—was both daunting and exhilarating. It lit a fire in me to keep pushing forward.

The grants focused on amplifying BIPOC and Queer voices in Appalachia and bridging Kentucky's rural-urban divide. With that funding, I launched *Backwoods Literary Press*, an initiative to reclaim and document narratives from rural communities, small towns, and reservations. In November 2024, we published *Discarded: A Rural Anthology*, featuring 63 artists from 27 states. The book captures a tapestry of experiences, from poetry rich in imagery to challenges against distorted urban stereotypes of rural America. Themes include discussions around Queerness, Christianity, colonialism, racism, and rural identity.

In just six months, I managed to establish a fiscally sponsored nonprofit, compile the works of 63 artists, and publish an anthology. The response has been overwhelmingly positive. We've sold enough to sustain the press and are preparing to publish another collection this year, with submissions opening in late spring. For updates, visit www.backwoodsliterarypress.com or follow us on Instagram at @backwoodsliterarypress.

This journey has taught me that being an artist isn't about financial success or formal accolades. It's about dedication to your craft and the courage to share your voice, even when it feels like no one is listening. The support I've received from organizations that uplift rural and Queer voices has been transformative, and I want to pay it forward by sharing these resources with others.

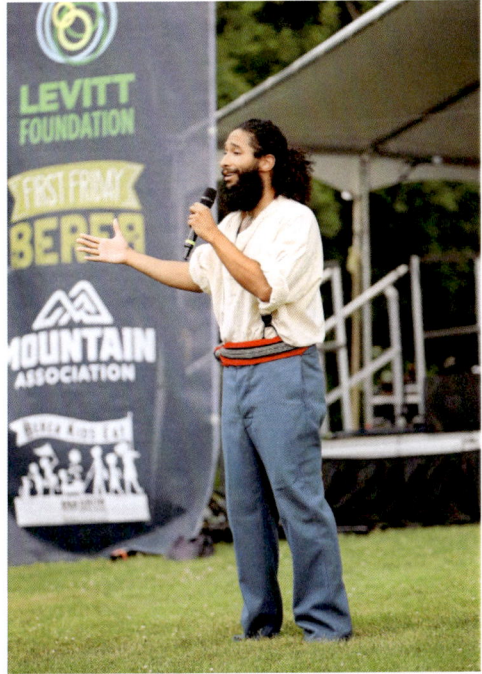

AFFRILACHIAN ARTS INSTITUTE, BEREA

Pictured, top left

www.affrilachianarts.org

Founded by Malcolm Davis, this institute uplifts Black artists in Appalachia by combining history and creative practice. Upcoming projects include performances at the Smithsonian Folklife Festival and a growing roster of Black Appalachian artists.

APPALSHOP, WHITESBURG

www.appalshop.org

Appalshop is a cultural cornerstone in Kentucky, using education, media, theater, and music to document and revitalize Appalachian traditions. It challenges stereotypes, supports justice, and participates in global dialogue. Notable works include the documentaries *I Know My Body* and *As Long As You Can*, which explore Queer experiences in Appalachia.

ARTMARKIT, COVINGTON

Pictured, bottom left

www.artmarkitcov.com

ArtMarkit, a Queer-owned creative hub in Northern Kentucky, offers access to gently used art supplies, mentorship, and workshops. It aims to make creative expression accessible and provides space for community engagement and artistic growth.

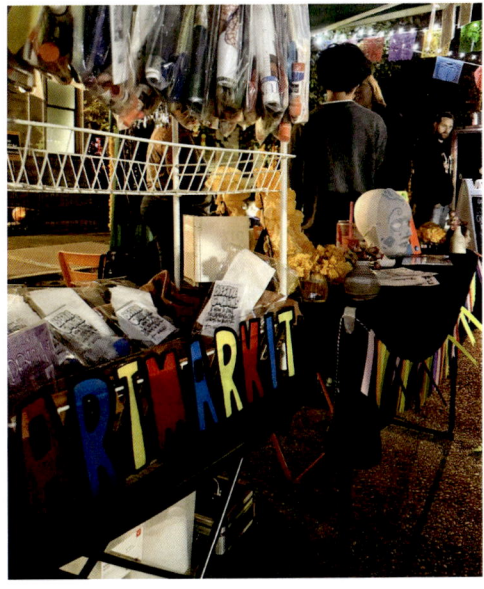

1. Malcolm Davis, photo courtesy of Affrilachian Arts Institute
2. Photo courtesy of Artmarkit

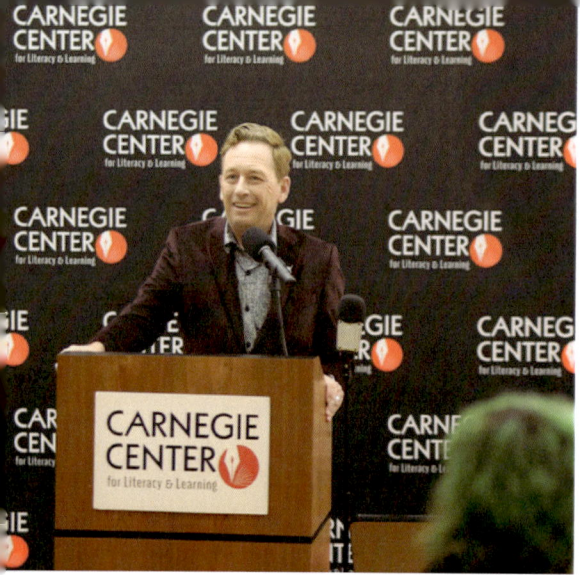

PRISM AREA ARTS ALLIANCE, OWENSBORO

www.prismartsalliance.org

Based in Western Kentucky, the Prism Arts Alliance promotes Queer expression in Daviess County. It provides a safe space for Queer people to express themselves artistically, with weekly meetups for actors, writers, artists, and poets.

CARNEGIE CENTER FOR LITERACY AND LEARNING, LEXINGTON

Pictured, left

www.carnegiecenterlex.org

The Carnegie Center offers classes in writing, publishing, and languages, as well as outreach programs and literary events. Many programs are free or have scholarships available. It celebrates LGBTQIA+ diversity through events like Queer author panels and the Queer Literary Hoedown, with a zero-tolerance policy for discrimination.

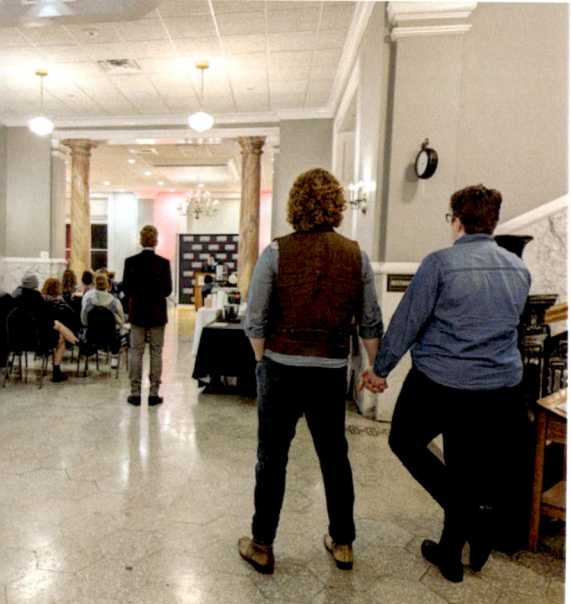

GATEWAY REGIONAL ARTS CENTER (GRAC), MT. STERLING

www.grackentucky.org

GRAC believes in "all the arts for all the people," connecting the landscapes and cultures of Central and Eastern Kentucky through various art forms. They host the Small Town America Institute for Rural Arts & Culture, which supports rural arts councils with resources and research to enhance community vibrancy.

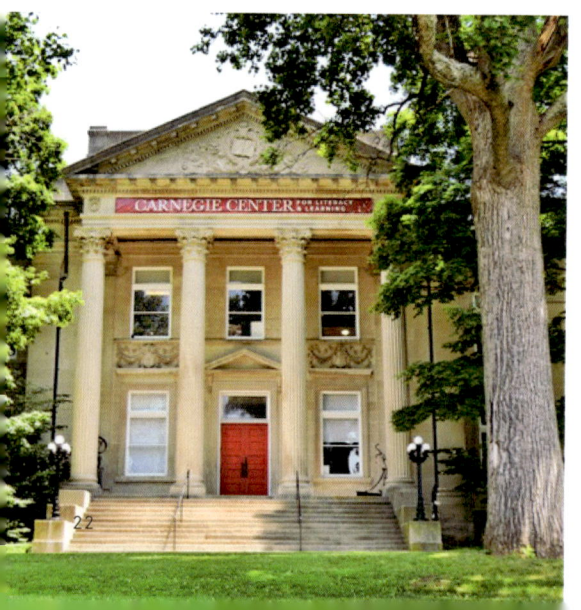

1. *Silas House, photo courtesy of Carnegie Center*
2. *Photo courtesy of Carnegie Center*
3. *Photo courtesy of GRAC*

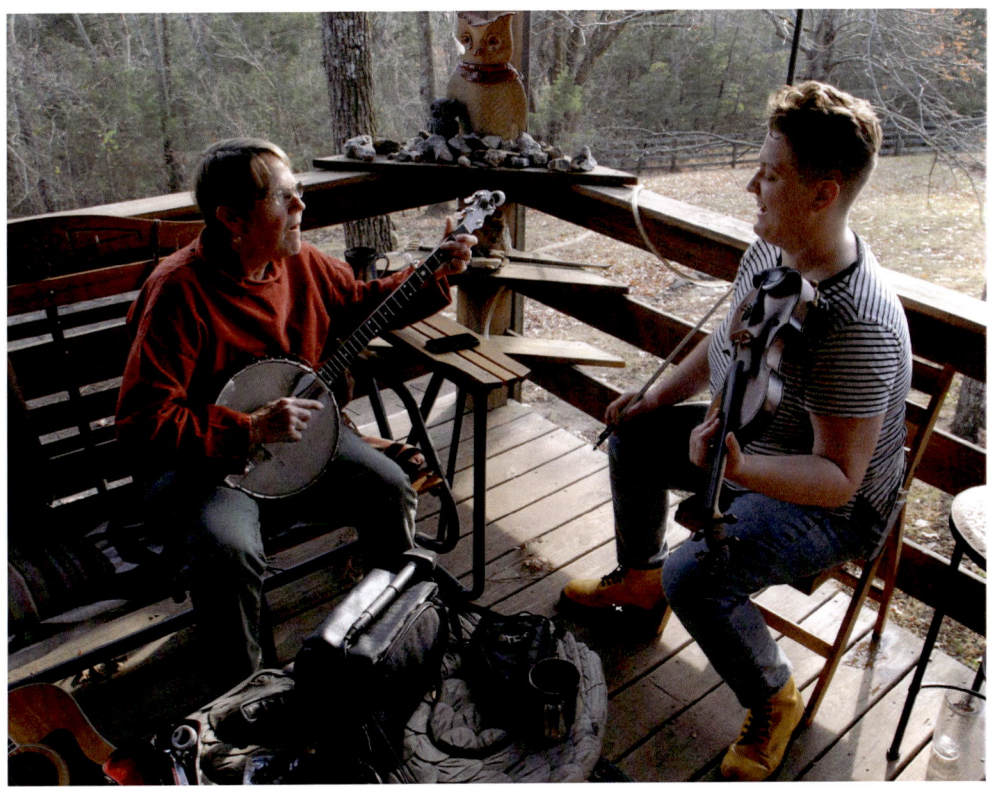

KENTUCKY ARTS COUNCIL, STATEWIDE

Pictured above

www.artscouncil.ky.gov

The Kentucky Arts Council supports artists across the state with grants and programs like the Al Smith Fellowship, Emerging Artist Program, and others. It also offers the Kentucky Peer Advisory Network, where professionals provide free consultations on areas like grant writing, marketing, and strategic planning. The Kentucky Arts Partnership Grant Program supports arts organizations with operating funding.

In conclusion, my journey as an artist has been centered around discovery, resilience, and the power of community. I have learned that being an artist is not defined by financial success or formal accolades, but by the commitment to craft and the willingness to share your voice, regardless of if you have an audience or not. Through collaboration and support from organizations that uplift rural and Queer voices, I have not only found my own path, but a collective strength in working together to create more inclusive spaces for diverse creators. Together, we can bridge divides, amplify voices pushed to the margin, and continue to develop Kentucky's artistic landscape. To fellow artists: pursue your craft, connect with your community, and remember that your voice is needed—now more than ever.

Sue Massek (left) and Larah Helayne (right) play the banjo and fiddle together. photo courtesy of Kentucky Arts Council

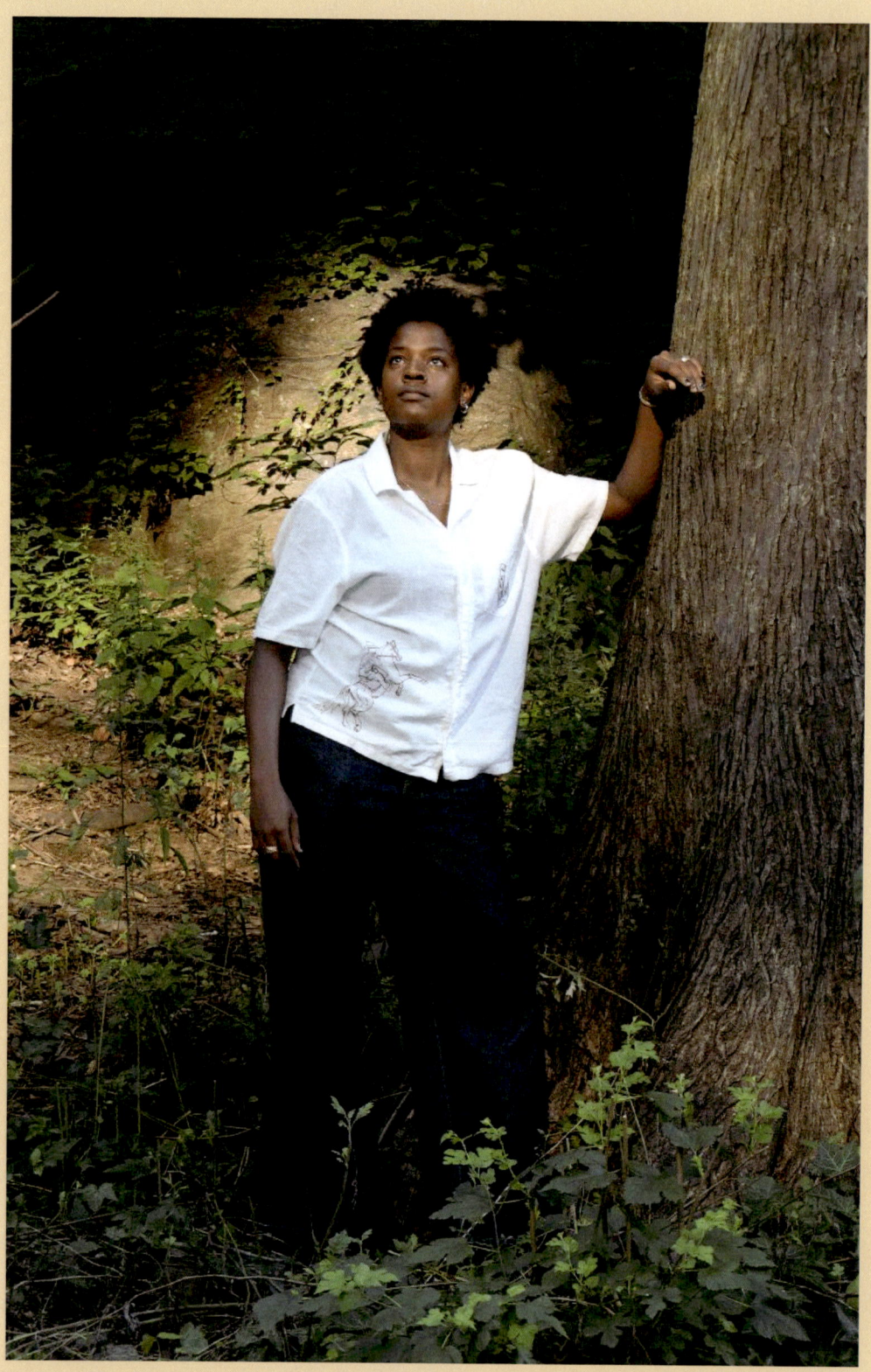

PERFORMANCE AS RESISTANCE

Imani N. Dennison she/they @imaninikyah

Identity is not static. It is a dynamic process, shaped by the spaces we occupy and the relationships we form. In many ways, life itself is a performance. We adapt, survive, and navigate our existence through acts of expression—often without fully realizing the weight of our roles. For me, as a Black Queer Southerner, performance has always been both a survival mechanism and a pathway to self-discovery. It is a practice that allows me to better understand who I am and, perhaps more importantly, who I am becoming. Love, in its truest form, emerges from this ongoing process of understanding—recognizing not only the selves we project to the world but also those we keep hidden or are still learning to embrace. It is messy, imperfect, and ever-evolving, but it is also what drives me forward. In those moments when doubt and uncertainty threaten to take hold, I remember: the show must go on!

As a multidisciplinary artist and filmmaker, my work grapples with the intricacies of personal history, memory, and the legacies of folklore. Performance, in this context, is both an act of defiance and an assertion of presence. It is a method of reclaiming space in a world that was never designed for us. And yet, the creative process often invites doubt. Imposter syndrome lurks at the edges, questioning my right to claim these stories and inhabit these roles. But in these moments, I feel the presence of my ancestors—those who, through their own performances of survival, carved paths for me to walk. Storytelling, I am reminded, is not a privilege, but a birthright. Each story I tell, each frame I create, is an act of resistance to erasure, a refusal to remain invisible. To create is to insist on the value of our narratives, to recognize the complexity of our existence, and to pass down the histories that demand to be carried forward.

Images by Jeremy Grier   he/him   @jeregrier

TO PERFORM IS TO SURVIVE, TO TRANSFORM, TO ADAPT.

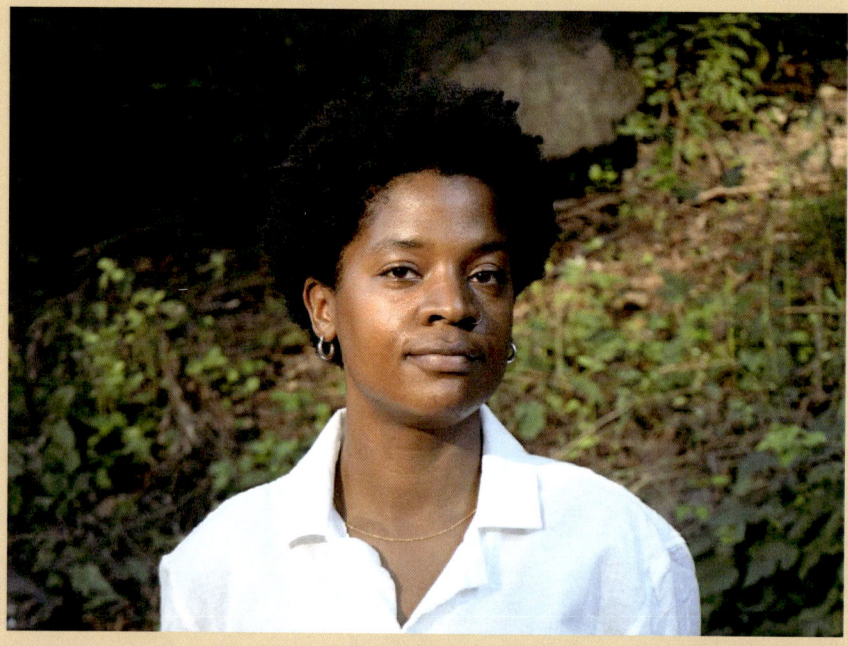

Recovery, too, is a performance—a quiet, often invisible act of reassembling what has been broken. To survive in a world that has consistently rejected your humanity is an act of performance in itself. It is an act of endurance. It is the performance of not allowing them to see you falter—of putting on the mask of hope, of code-switching to navigate spaces that were thoughtfully built in your opposition. There are times when the body speaks louder than the will. There are moments when there is no energy left for pretending, no capacity for performance. In those moments, we must lean into the complexity of grief, of exhaustion—because to heal, we must stop the show. We must stop to listen to our bodies, to honor the fullness of our emotions, and to embrace the radical necessity of rest. This pause is not surrender; it is a radical act of self-care and restoration that enables us to return with renewed strength.

In the pauses between performances, I have learned to rely on my Queer kin. It is they who have taught me how to find joy in the cracks, how to dance in the rain, even when despair threatens to swallow us whole. It is through them that I understand that even in the most difficult of times, there is always space to breathe, to move, to begin again. To perform is to survive, to transform, to adapt. It is how we make sense of the fragments of our lives, how we turn brokenness into story, and stories into futures. Each performance, each gesture, each moment of self-expression is a declaration: we are here. And when the show must stop—when we are compelled to rest, to breathe, to heal—let that be an act of radical care. The show must go on, but it is in the pauses, in the moments of stillness, that we gather the strength to keep moving forward!

proudly designed by BRACKISH *a branding studio*
www.brackishcreative.com

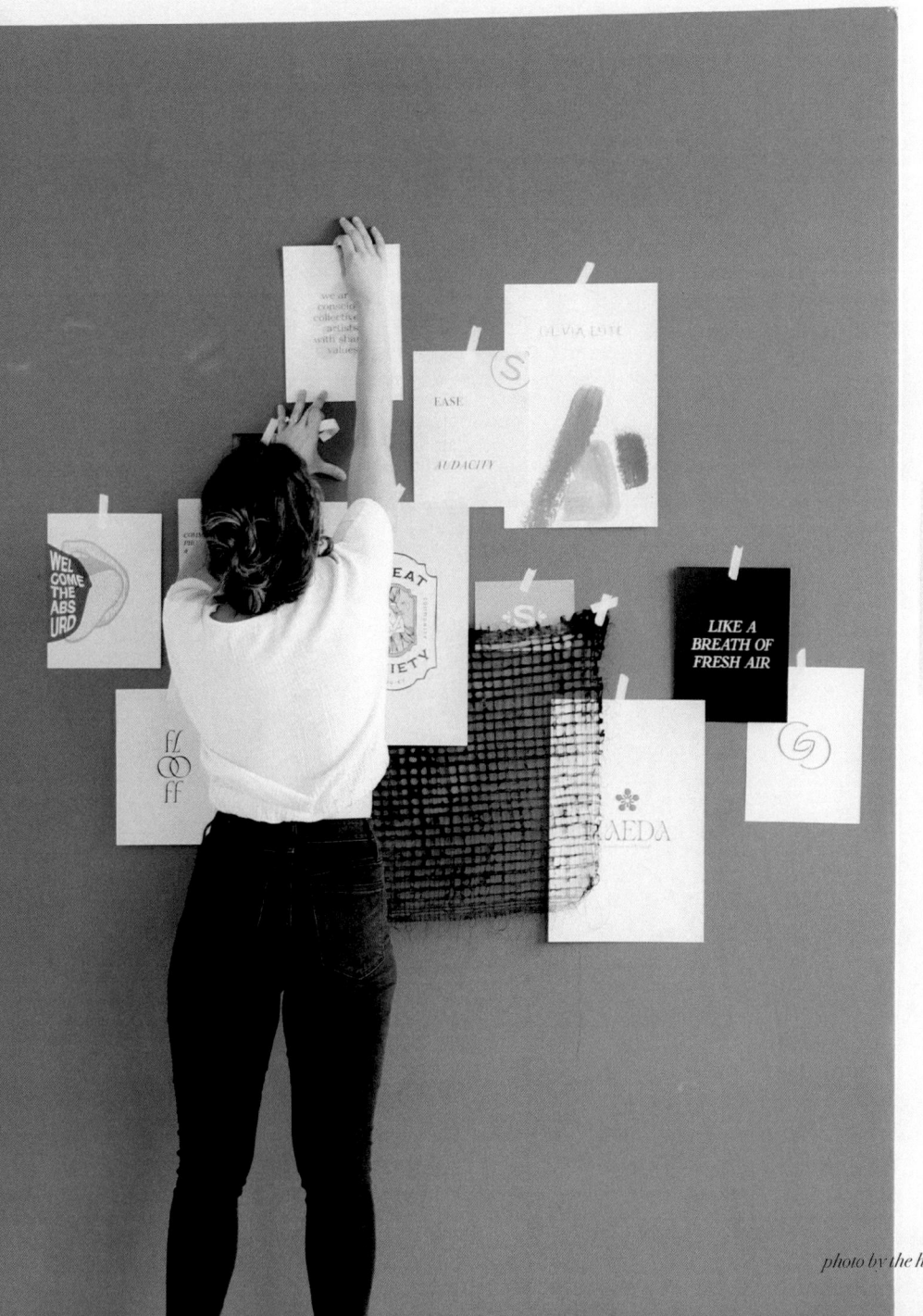

photo by the humble lion

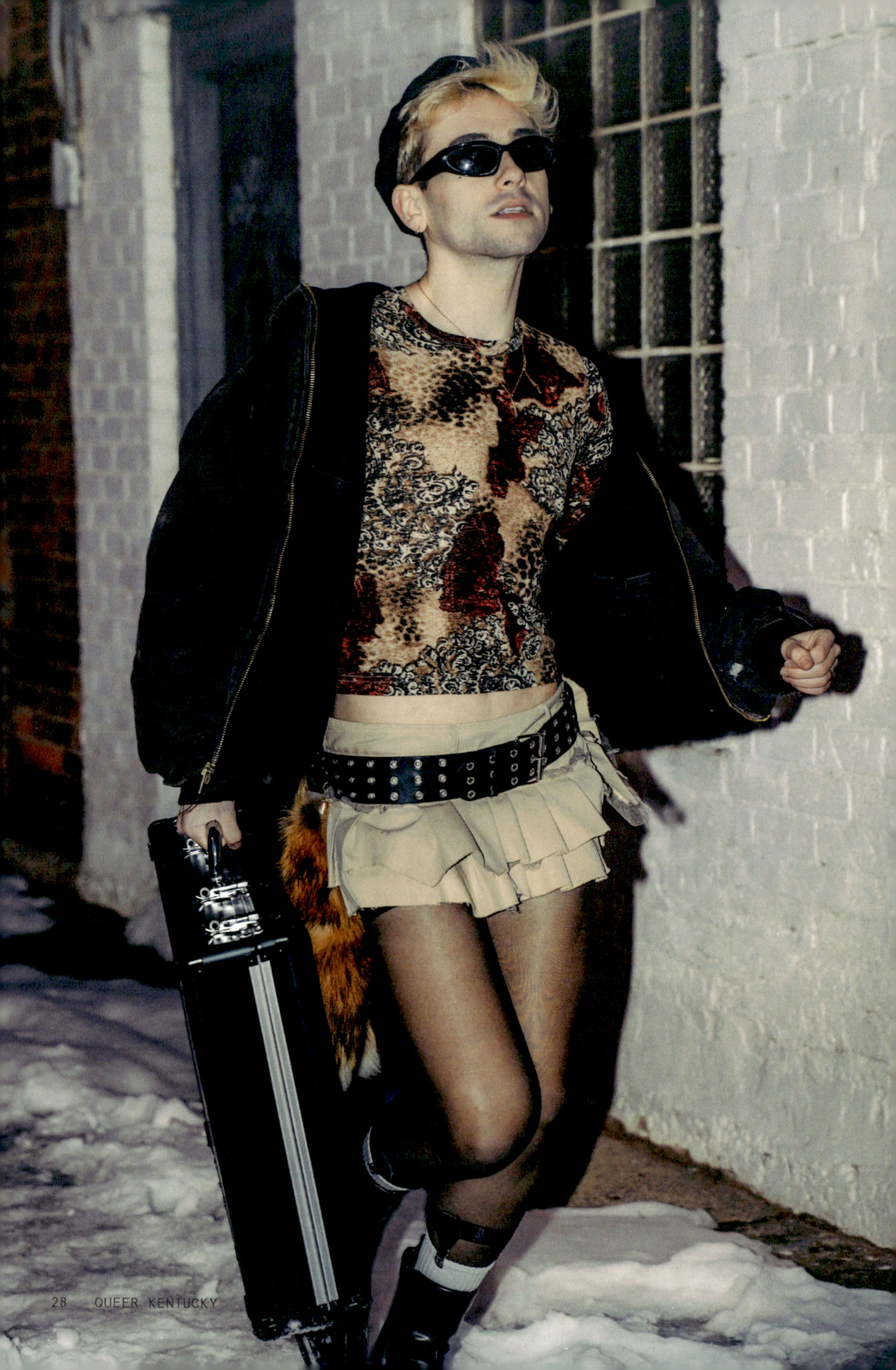

AN INTERVIEW WITH DJ BOYWIFE

QUEEN OUT OR GET OUT

Spencer Jenkins *he/him @spencerjenkss*

SUMMER 2024, DUBBED POP GIRLY SUMMER, OR "BRAT" SUMMER BY THE QUEERS, INSPIRED BY CHARLI XCX'S SUMMER RELEASE OF THE SAME NAME, BROUGHT THE RISE OF THE MIDWEST PRINCESS CHAPPELL ROAN, A TASTE OF ESPRESSO FROM BLONDE BOMBSHELL SABRINA CARPENTER, AND ONE "CLUB, CLUB CLASSIC" BUMPING DJ WHO WAS CROWNED THE NEWEST IT-GIRL OF THE OHIO RIVER VALLEY.

DJ Boywife, or Shane Brouman, 27, Hebron, is an openly Queer person, with an affinity for black micro miniskirts, espresso martinis, and creating Queer- and trans-affirming experiences focused around tearing up a dancefloor to what he dubs as the "faggiest" of music.

"Kim Petra's 'Slut Pop?' Yes, please!" he says while sipping his martini across from me at Alice Bar in the Over the Rhine neighborhood of Cincinnati.

The blonde pixie-esque cut club kid with Julia Fox painted eyes could resemble any main character out of the 2003 cult classic, *Party Monster*—the true crime story where McCauley Culkin portrays the club promoter and convicted murderer, Micahel Alig. Parallels between Alig and Brauman exist in their Queer campy personae and how they became catalysts to Queer counterculture club movements, but Brauman could only ever murder on the dance floor.

"I need to see people dancing and having a good time, or I feel like I'm not doing my job," he says. "If you're not dancing, you're taking up space for someone who maybe would enjoy it and you're sucking the energy out of the room."

He went on to discuss the difference between pre- and post-pandemic club behavior. Brauman noted that his dance floor might very well be someone's first.

"A lot of the people who come to dance turned 21 during the pandemic and never had the chance to experience clubbing like others did," he says. "You can listen to pop girl music at home, but it hits differently when you're dancing body to body. I love seeing people experience music that way. Charli doesn't call it 'home home classics.' She said, 'Club, club!'"

Even for those of us who aren't so freshly coming-of-age and entering the club scene, a DJ Boywife show feels like being around gay people for the first time. You feel seen and understood, like you can finally exhale. Whether it's the light and laser projections around the room, or the bass shaking through your chest, the air is thick with joy.

And then the music is inevitable. It's less of a choice to dance, and more of an unstoppable force that pulls you to the dance floor and keeps you there as each song somehow gets better than the last. It's a space where everyone is in on the same secret: that, for just a few hours, you can put on some lipstick and eyeliner and let your girly boy out. Nothing matters but the freedom to just be.

For someone who creates these magnetic spaces with such seeming ease, Brouman never planned to become the—

> "OH MY GOD, ARE YOU DJ BOYFWIFE?" she cried, eyes wide, appearing from whatever dark place fans originate. "You won't remember me, but I danced around the entire Queen City Radio Bar during your set and was explaining the cultural significance of Sabrina Carpenter's *Bed Chem* to everyone around me. ANYWAYS, I LOVE YOU."

And off she went, back to the fan-depths from whence she came.

"I paid her to do that specifically for this interview," Brauman jokingly laughs. "I can't walk into a bathroom without seeing 'I love DJ Boywife' graffiti on the wall, which is highly rewarding."

Brouman never planned to become the Boywife he is today. His journey into DJing started by chance at a friend's going-away party, where a promoter pointed at him and said, "You should DJ—you look like a DJ." It wasn't until he started bumping his favorite Sophie tracks behind the booth that he slipped on his first pair of heels and pleather mini, fully embracing the persona that now defines his sets.

"I didn't wear makeup when I first started DJing, but I fell into it and it felt natural," he tells me. "I don't have the story of putting on my mom's heels and stuff, but drag queens would lend me clothes to wear, and I just love wearing them. It's not a Boywife set if I'm not wearing a micromini. Being a gay kid growing up in Ohio, the opportunity to feel sexy and confident was scarce," he says. "When I started DJing I felt more eyes on me and I thought 'Why don't I show off?' I worked for it."

The Sophie stanning DJ rose from performing at small venues in Cincinnati to becoming a

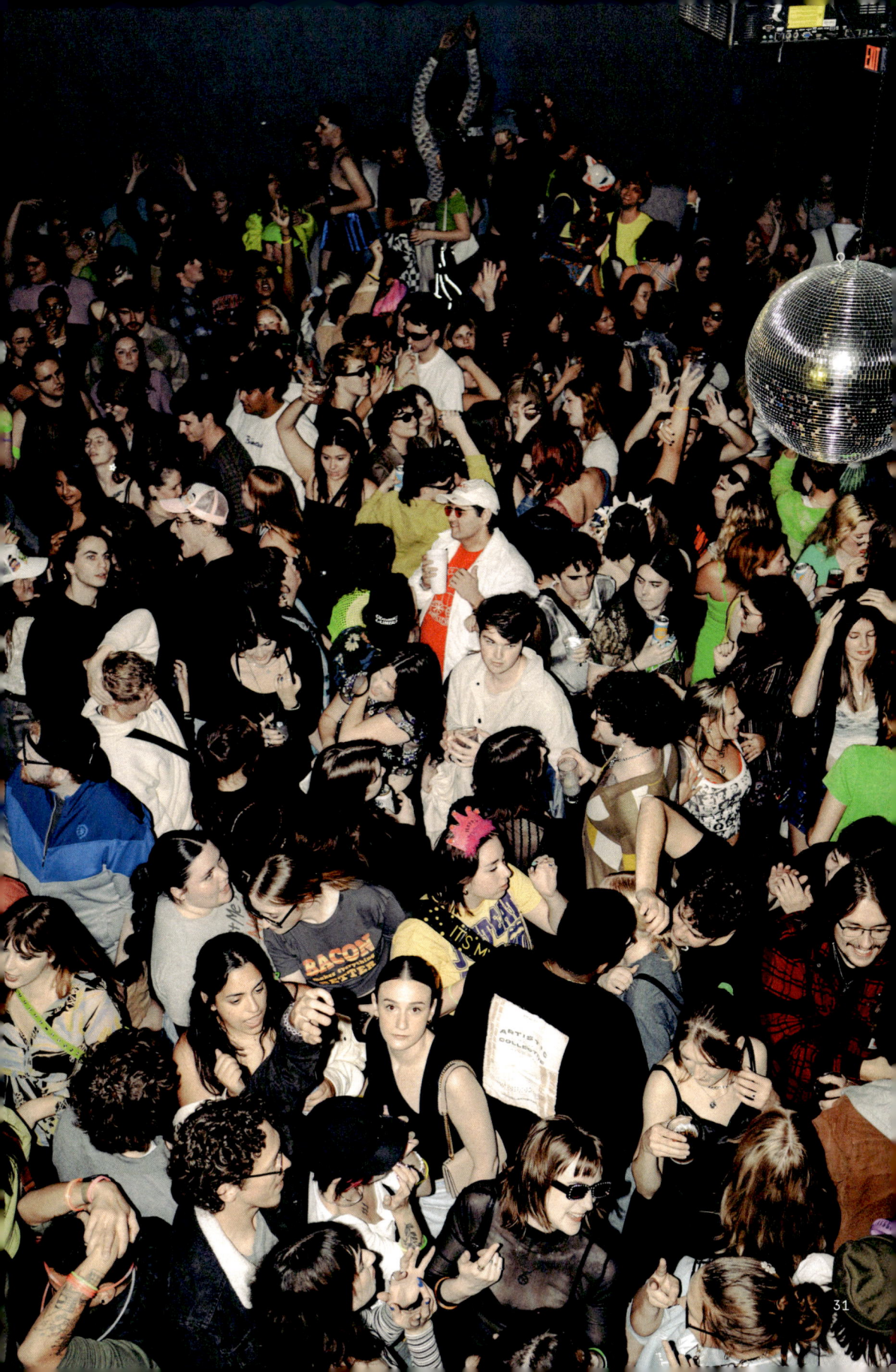

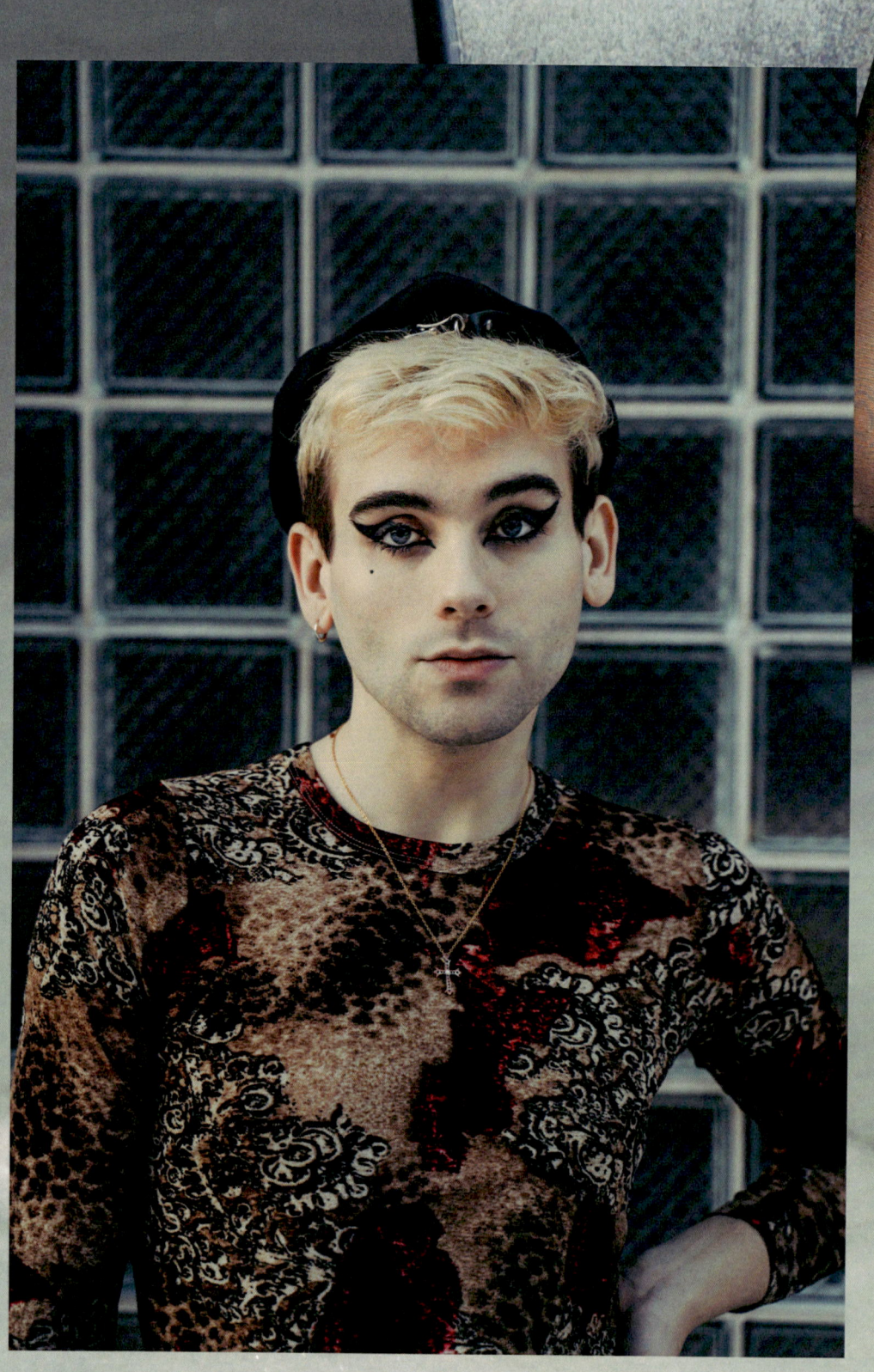

OH MY GOD, ARE YOU DJ BOYFWIFE?

resident DJ at some of the city's larger spots. He has also booked gigs across Kentucky and Ohio, including a standout New Year's Eve show with Rebecca Black at Cincinnati's Hard Rock Cafe.

Creating a Queer- and trans-affirming vibe is of utmost importance to Brouman, but it isn't always easy, especially when the venue isn't strictly a Queer-only space. Brouman is the resident DJ at Alice, which has a mixed crowd of gays, theys, and straights. But when Brouman's set begins, the room has no choice but to queen out or get out.

"Truly sometimes it's the straight guys begging to hear Kim Petra's "Treat Me Like A Slut," he laughs. "Like my sets get so gay no matter what."

At the beginning of each set he shouts on the mic, "Who's gay? Who's trans?'" setting the space up for Queer vibes only. He says he has received messages from trans folks telling them that no one's ever asked "who is trans" at a club they've attended, making them feel seen and heard.

"It blows my mind. That's the DJ's job—to create a space where everyone feels seen and celebrated," he said. "I'm always going to cater to the Queer community and I love and support the trans community so much because they've done so much for me in my life. Of course I'm going to uplift their existence during my set," he said.

He notes that he wouldn't be doing what he loves if it weren't for the inspiration of trans DJ Louisville legend, DJ Syimone.

"Trans people are everything and DJ Syimone is so fierce and I love her," he says. "Also, If I could, I would only make music for trans people. If I were only DJing for gay cis people and straights, I would have to quit DJing."

In a Boywife world, trans people are always winning, and he says that's what he wants to see in 2025 — trans joy and freedom. The freedom to love and exist fully on his dance floor.

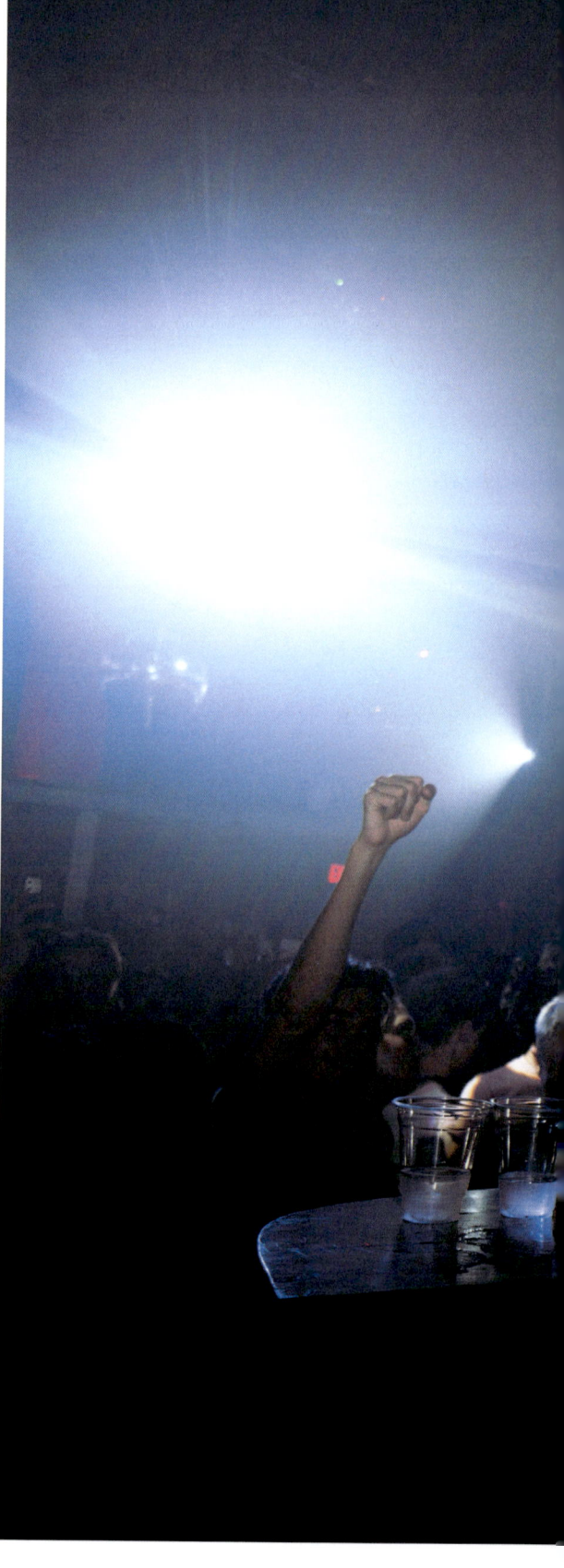

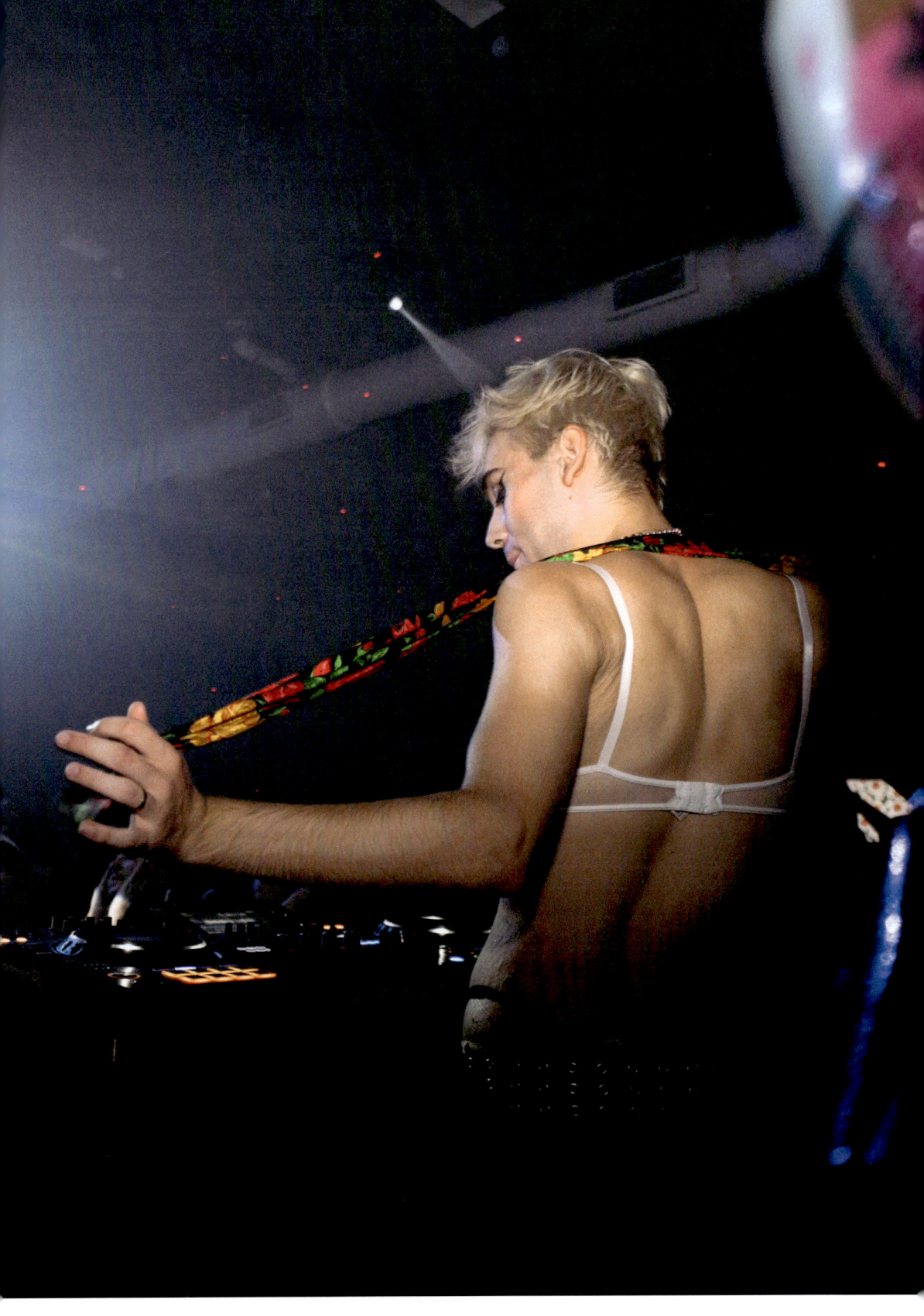

The Best Gay One-Night Stand in America

PERFORMING IN LEXINGTON, 1970S-1980S

Faulkner Morgan Archive *@faulknermorganarchive*

Divine performing at Club Au Go Go, photo by Jim Shauffer, January 28, 1982, Collection of Faulkner Morgan Archive.

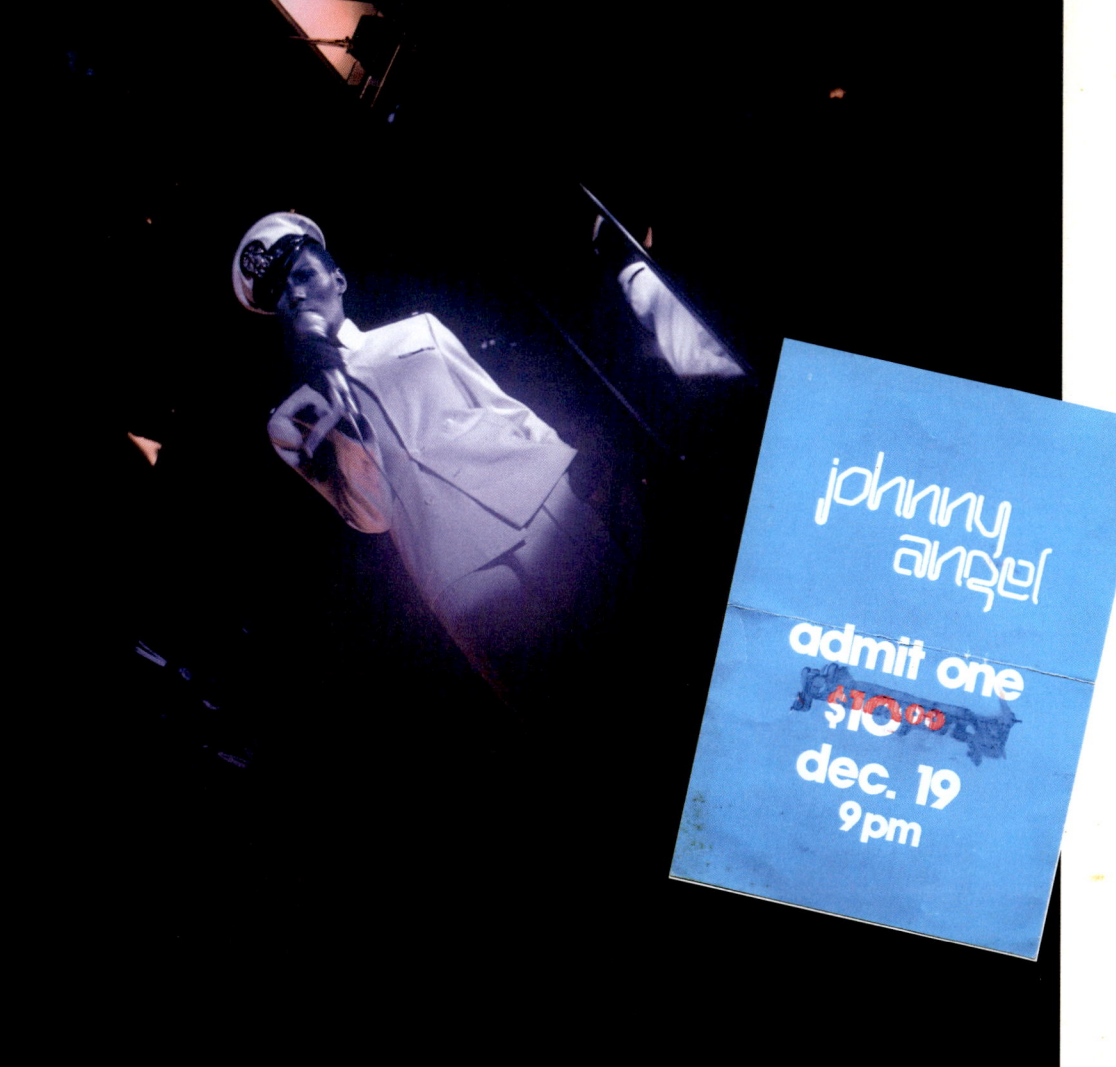

Ticket to see *Grace Jones* at Johnny Angel, December 19, 1978, collection of Faulkner Morgan Archive.
Grace Jones performing at Johnny Angel, photo by Melissa Watt, December 19, 1978

For one night and one night only, Lexington hosted some of the most visibly Queer entertainers of the 1970s and 1980s. Drawn by the city's reputation as a gay haven, and facilitated by the connections of several bar owners, Lexington became a "one-night stand" as celebrities stopped to perform on their way to other, larger cities.

Lexington being renowned as a "one-night stand" city for performers, though, was nothing new. During the 19th and early 20th centuries, Lexington was a popular stop on the theatrical touring circuit for famous actors and actresses, as explained by author Kevin Lane Dearinger in his 2023 lecture, "The Best One-Night Stand in America: The Rich Theatrical History of Lexington, 1808-1918." While the rise of movie theaters eventually caused Lexington's reputation as the "best one-night stand to fade," Queer venues and bars later served a similar function by bringing popular entertainers to Kentucky.

Just months after opening in 1978, Johnny Angel, located at 224 East Main Street, brought Grace Jones to their "million-dollar dance floor" designed by the creators of New York City's infamous Studio 54. The bar was filled with patrons excited to witness Jones during her rise as an icon of the gay disco scene.

THE SHOW MUST GO ON

John Davis, the manager of Johnny Angel, recalled details of that night in an interview with Faulkner Morgan Archive. He remembered how Jones was transported in a 1954 Rolls Royce, which broke down on the way to her hotel room. The Herald-Leader covered the event, but painted a bathing suit over Jones before running photographs of her. She undressed men and women during her act. One was a young construction worker who was bribed by Christian Jones—Grace's gay brother—to let her strip him down to just a jockstrap by the time the show was over.

Grace Jones wasn't the only disco icon to grace the dance floor of 224 East Main. The legendary Sylvester performed to an ecstatic audience in 1984. When Sylvester arrived to do a sound check, he was wearing a long fur overcoat and carrying a very large handbag. He walked upstairs, looked around, dropped the bag, and asked the DJ to put on one of the backing tracks so he could hear it over the system. Once the music came on, he let out one of his famous hollers and said, "That's fine. Let's go to the hotel."

Other stars who performed at Johnny Angel, and later The Bar Complex, included Debbie Jacobs, Linda Clifford, and Sally Kellerman. It wasn't just disco celebrities, though, that were attracted to the Bluegrass state. Another Queer icon that came to perform in Lexington was the infamous Divine. A "one-night stand," however, was clearly not enough for her. Divine visited Kentucky multiple times throughout her career and played Lexington several times in the 1980s while at the height of her fame.

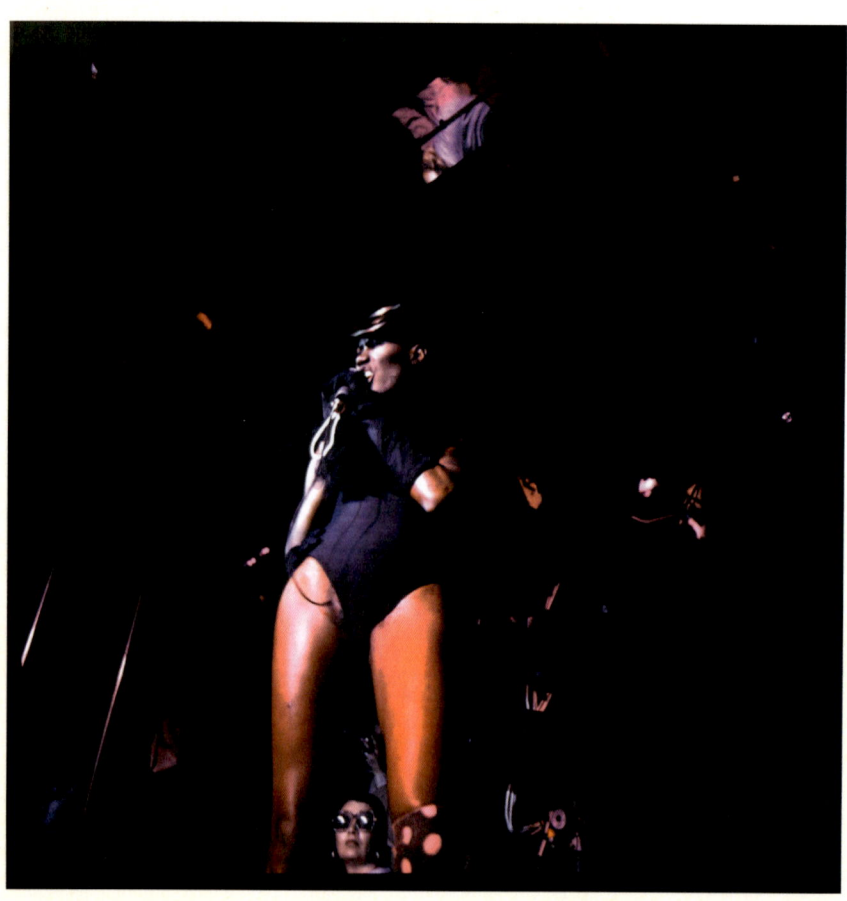

Grace Jones performing at Johnny Angel, photo by Melissa Watt, December 19, 1978, collection of Faulkner Morgan Archive.

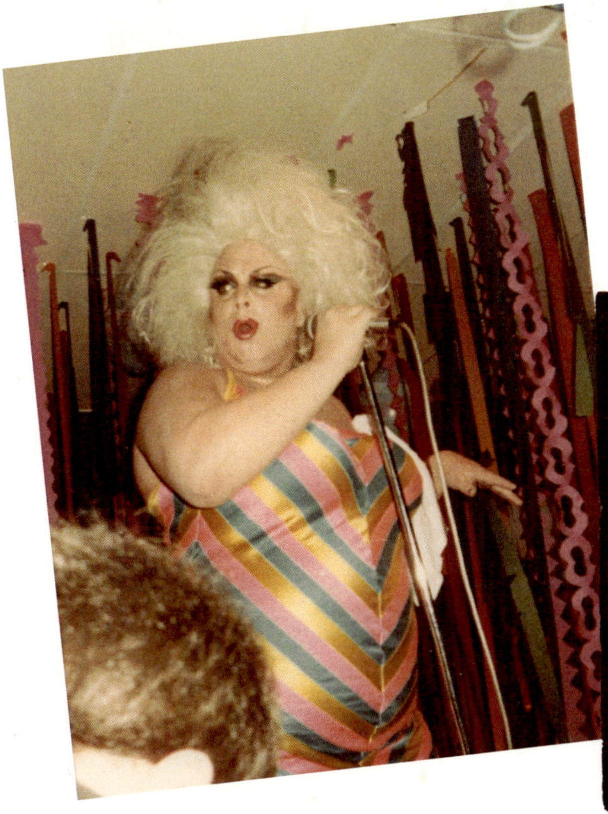

Divine performing at Club Au Go Go, photo by Jim Shauffer, January 28, 1982, Collection of Faulkner Morgan Archive.

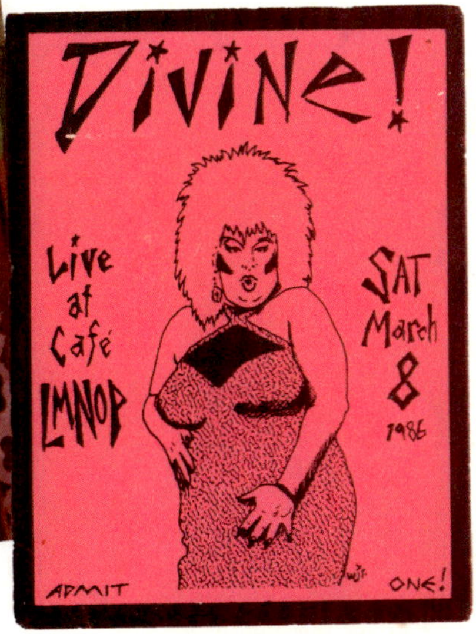

Ticket to see Divine at Café LMNOP, Designed by Bill Widener Jr., 1986, collection of Faulkner Morgan Archive.

Mostly eschewing small cities, Divine was lured to Lexington by its reputation for Queer decadence and her friendship with manager Bradley Picklesimer of Lexington's Club Au Go Go and Café LMNOP. She performed at the bars on January 28, 1982 and March 8, 1986, respectively. In a review of the show that was published in the *Kentucky Kernel*, a student newspaper at the University of Kentucky, Margo Ravel describes the performance as a "queen-sized dose of bad taste."

Club Au Go Go and Café LMNOP, were both known for hosting a plethora of underground and punk rock performers as well. This space gave the opportunities to bands both local and traveling. Some of the most notable bands included The Thrusters, Red Interiors, and Human Sexual Response.

While celebrities performing one-night-only gigs on the dance floors of Lexington's gay bars is not quite as common of an occurrence anymore, Kentucky as a whole still attracts many Queer icons to the bluegrass. From Chappell Roan performing at Kentuckiana Pride to the countless drag queens from *Rupaul's Drag Race* touring with Hard Candy Events, Kentucky is still a place for Queer decadence.

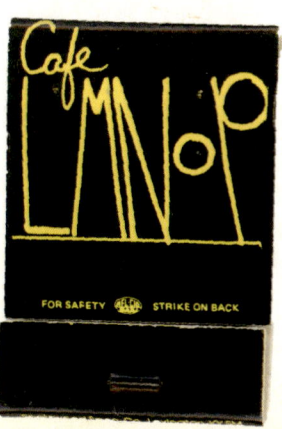

Café LMNOP matchbook, c. 1980s, collection of Faulkner Morgan Archive.

THE SHOW MUST GO ON

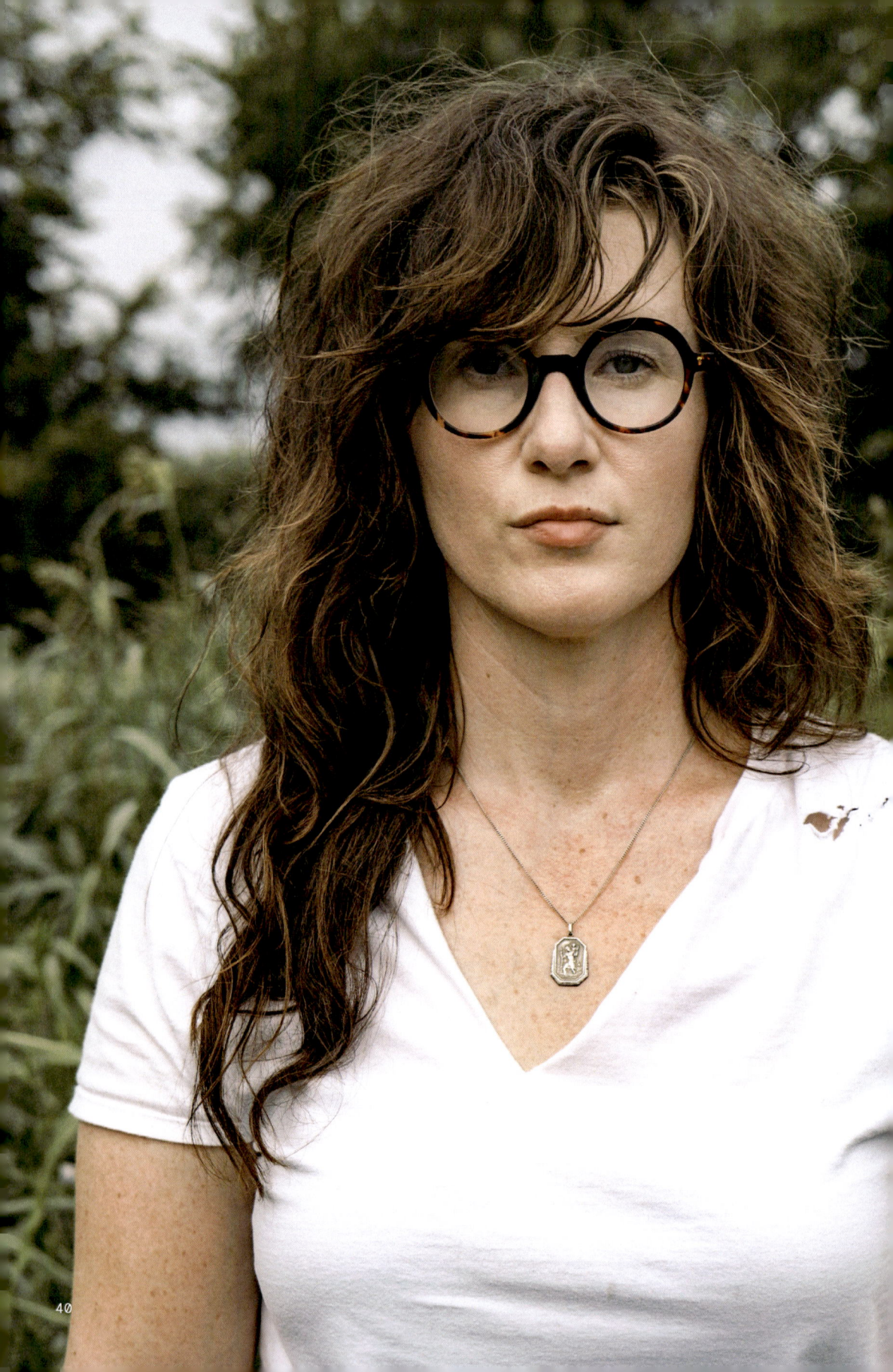

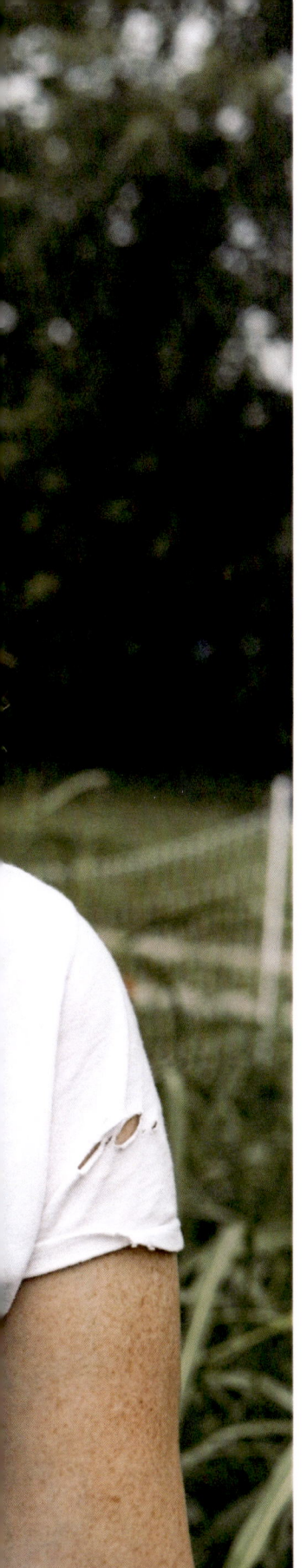

FROM NO STOPLIGHTS TO HER NAME IN LIGHTS
THE RISE OF S.G. GOODMAN

Belle Townsend they/she   @belletownsendky

Born in western Tennessee and raised across state lines in Hickman, Kentucky, S.G. Goodman's journey as an artist is deeply rooted in the landscape and culture of her upbringing. Hickman, a small town nestled in Fulton County along the Mississippi River, shaped much of her perspective. "I come from a long line of farmers. Hickman is a very small town. We didn't have fast food. We didn't have a stoplight. I'm ever finding out how much of an impact being raised in a rural, small community has had on me," she reflects.

Raised in the Southern Baptist church, Goodman credits her religious upbringing for some of her foundational skills as a musician. "I would consider myself a recovering Southern Baptist at this point in my life," she says with a hint of humor, but her reverence for the musical traditions of her childhood is clear. "Being that I've never had any formal training in music, I consider my time going to church three times a week as my formal training. If you dig, you find you're in a deep, rich history of singing style and a culture that is very specific to your area."

Goodman's connection to Kentucky runs deeper than music. Her father's work as a farmer instilled in her a sense of place, a tie to the landscape and its lushness. "After traveling the United States so many times in a year, the thickness around here is what I miss the most—the lushness of the vegetation and animals," she explains. Her home, part of the Lower Mississippi Delta region, offers a unique blend of landscapes, from cypress trees to slough waters. These visuals are central to her identity, both as an artist and as a Queer person.

Images by Carey Neal Gough   she/her   @careynealgough

"When thinking about how the landscape and where I was raised affected my Queerness, I would say it's always been really important to me," Goodman says, while acknowledging this understanding has been an evolving process. "I wasn't 12 and walking around saying I'm a Kentucky Queer." For Goodman, Queer identity and rural identity can be complicated to hold together, but she is committed to representation. "Now that I am this version of myself, and secure in my identity as a Queer person, I understand how important it is for rural representation in Queer spaces."

Her early experience at Murray State University underscores her sense of being an outsider. Coming from Hickman, her first encounters with the busier streets of Murray felt overwhelming. "I remember driving around the town, and you know, there's stoplights and bigger intersections and things way different than my little tiny hometown of Hickman. I felt so alone and like I didn't know if I was meant to be there or not." She humorously recounts struggling with traffic laws, having learned to drive on a farm by the age of seven. "I knew how to drive, but I didn't know the laws."

These feelings of uncertainty extended into the early years of her music career. "I oftentimes say, 'I'm thinking of my grandparents, sharecroppers who only finished 6th grade, and I say that I'm carving out all the places in the world that were meant for them.' Sometimes I have to remind myself that this is really who I am and my truth."

Goodman's music often mirrors this personal and cultural complexity. Her first album, *Old Time Feeling*, carries a love for her homeland, while her second, *Teeth Marks*, offers an exploration of trauma and empathy. "As far as the music I've put out currently, if we focus on the theme of love throughout it, I would say that my record *Old Time Feeling*... really spoke of a love for a place. *Teeth Marks* was more of a look inward."

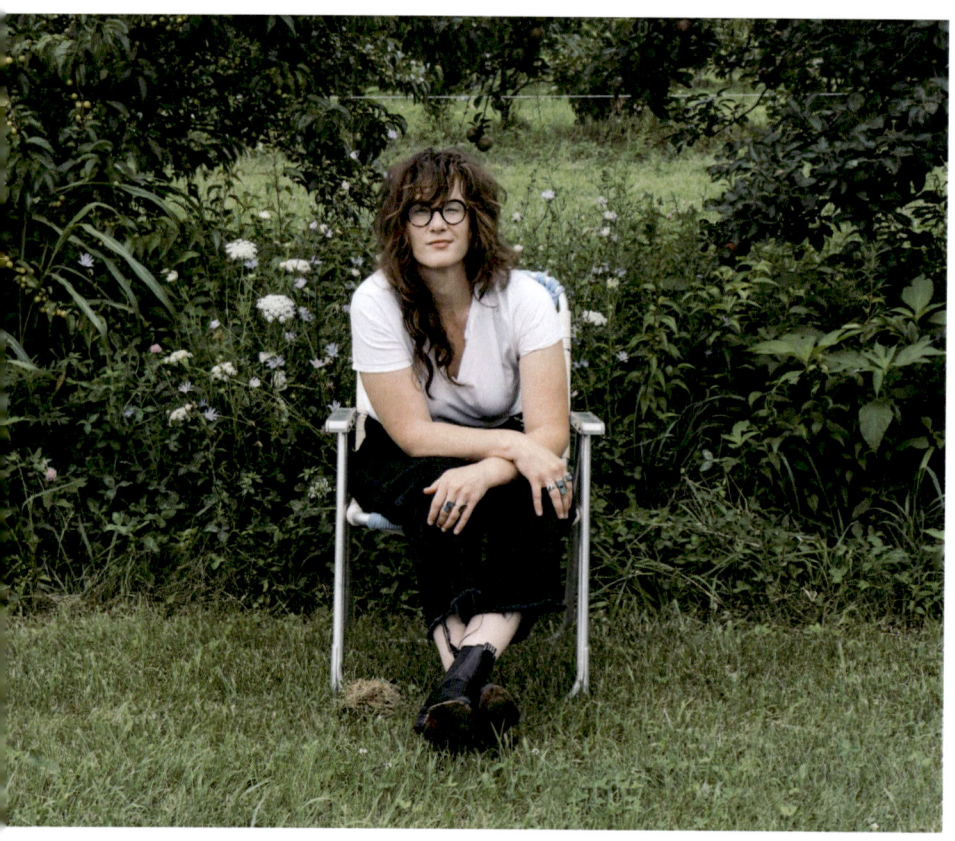

Her unique voice and evocative storytelling earned Goodman significant recognition, including the Emerging Artist of the Year award at the Americana Music Association Awards. Kentucky's first openly gay poet laureate and music journalist Silas House says, "S.G. is particularly important as a representative because she is completely herself in every way and she refuses to ever put aside her ruralness. It is a huge part of who she is, and especially the way that has shaped her in relation to her Queerness. Her music and her existence itself complexifies the notion of what it means to be a rural Queer person. I have tremendous respect for her music but also for who she is as an activist and as a representative for so many of us who don't see ourselves portrayed accurately in popular media enough."

Even as she finds success, Goodman wrestles with the complexity of her rural and Queer identities. "The only way to change a place is to stay put. And to do the work. And to live your life," she says, though she recognizes the nuance of that truth. She wants to believe it, but she understands that some people must leave for their safety or mental health. For Goodman, the tension between identity and geography is a story still unfolding, but it is one she tells with unflinching honesty and profound artistry.

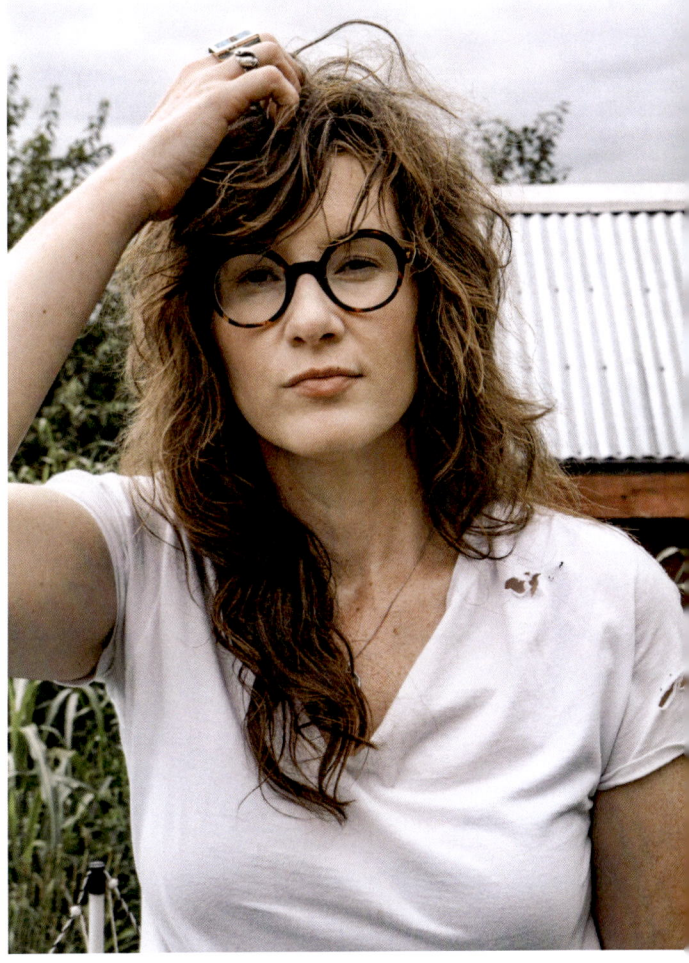

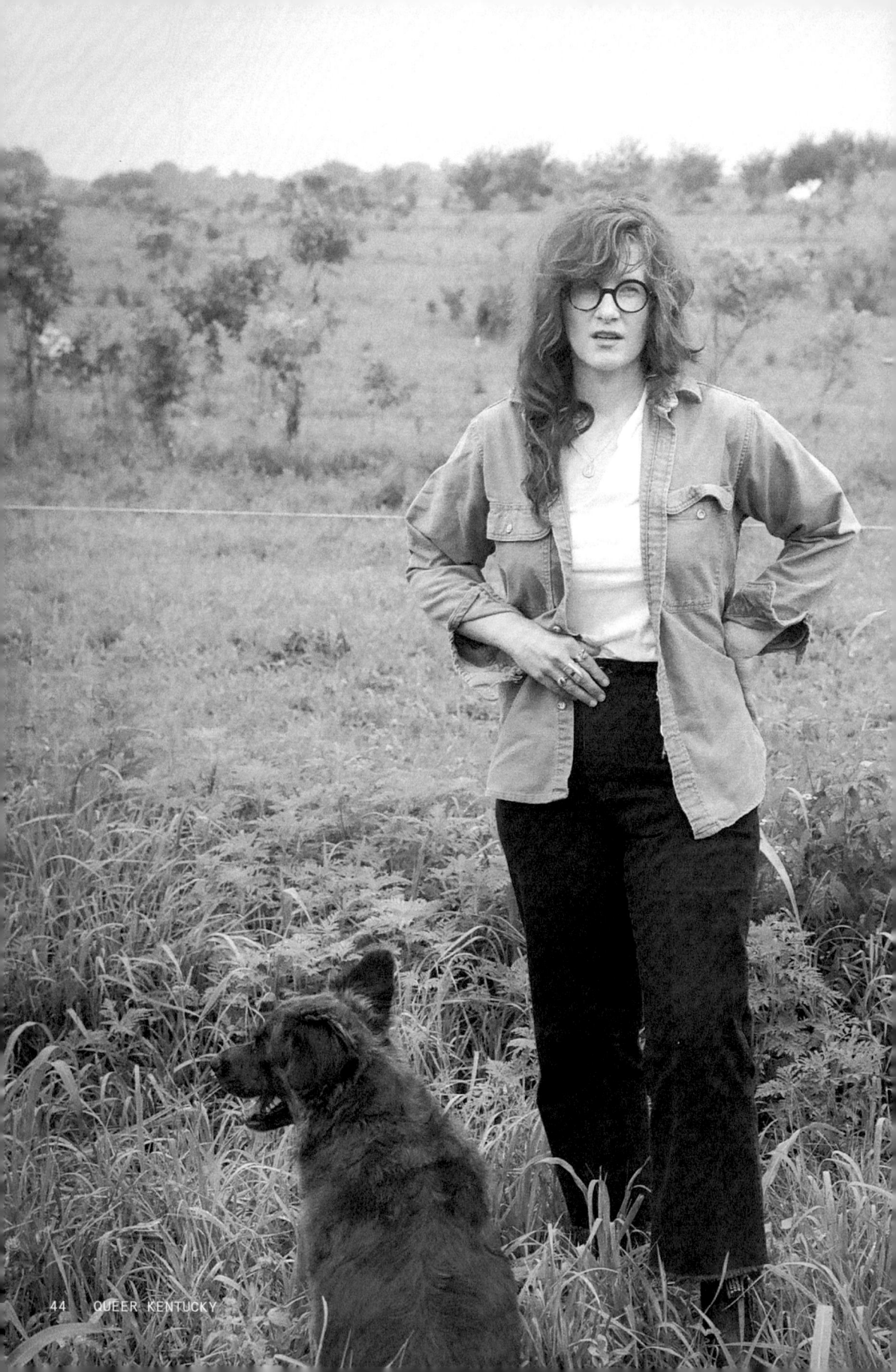

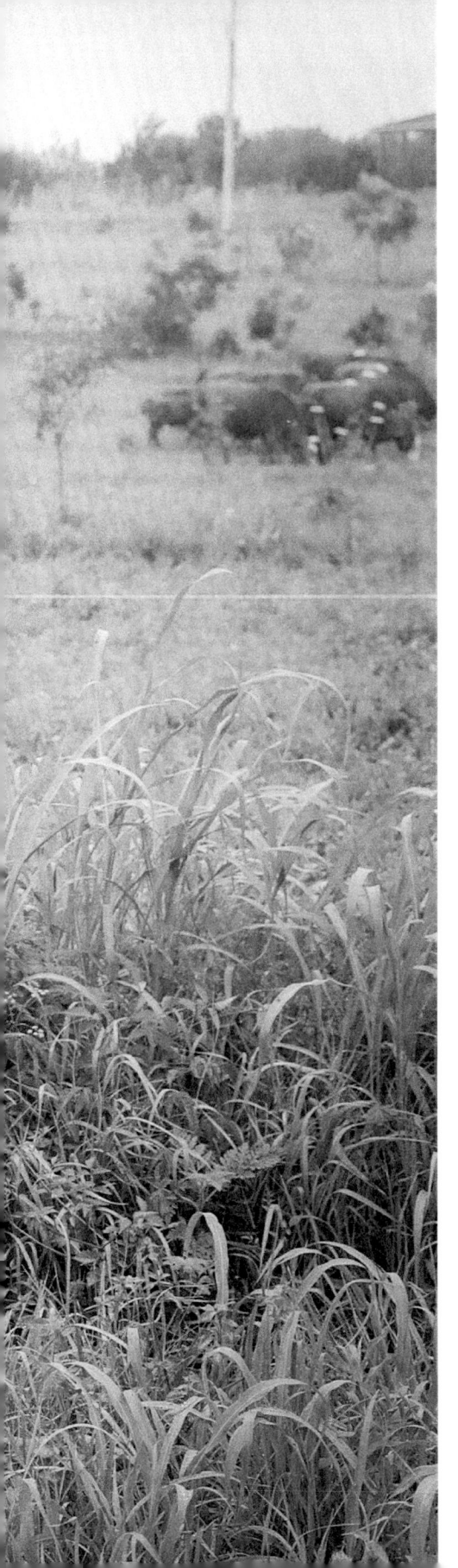

"THE ONLY WAY TO CHANGE A PLACE IS TO STAY PUT. AND TO DO THE WORK. AND TO LIVE YOUR LIFE."

BOONE COUNTY TO BARTSCHLAND

A LOOK INTO THE ANDREW DAHLING WORLD

Spencer Adkins he/him @therealspenceradkins

The last time I spoke with Andrew Dahling, the club kid diva from Boone County, his partnership as makeup artist to Chappell Roan was just beginning to take flight. Having done Roan's makeup at Governor's Ball, Bonnaroo, *The Tonight Show*, and the Kentuckiana Pride Festival, Dahling's career was at a tipping point. Since then, he's been as busy as ever painting the Midwest Princess and showing out at Bartschland in New York City. "It's been kind of a whirlwind," Dahling said of the past year.

Images by Alexey Kim he/she/they @sidewalkkilla

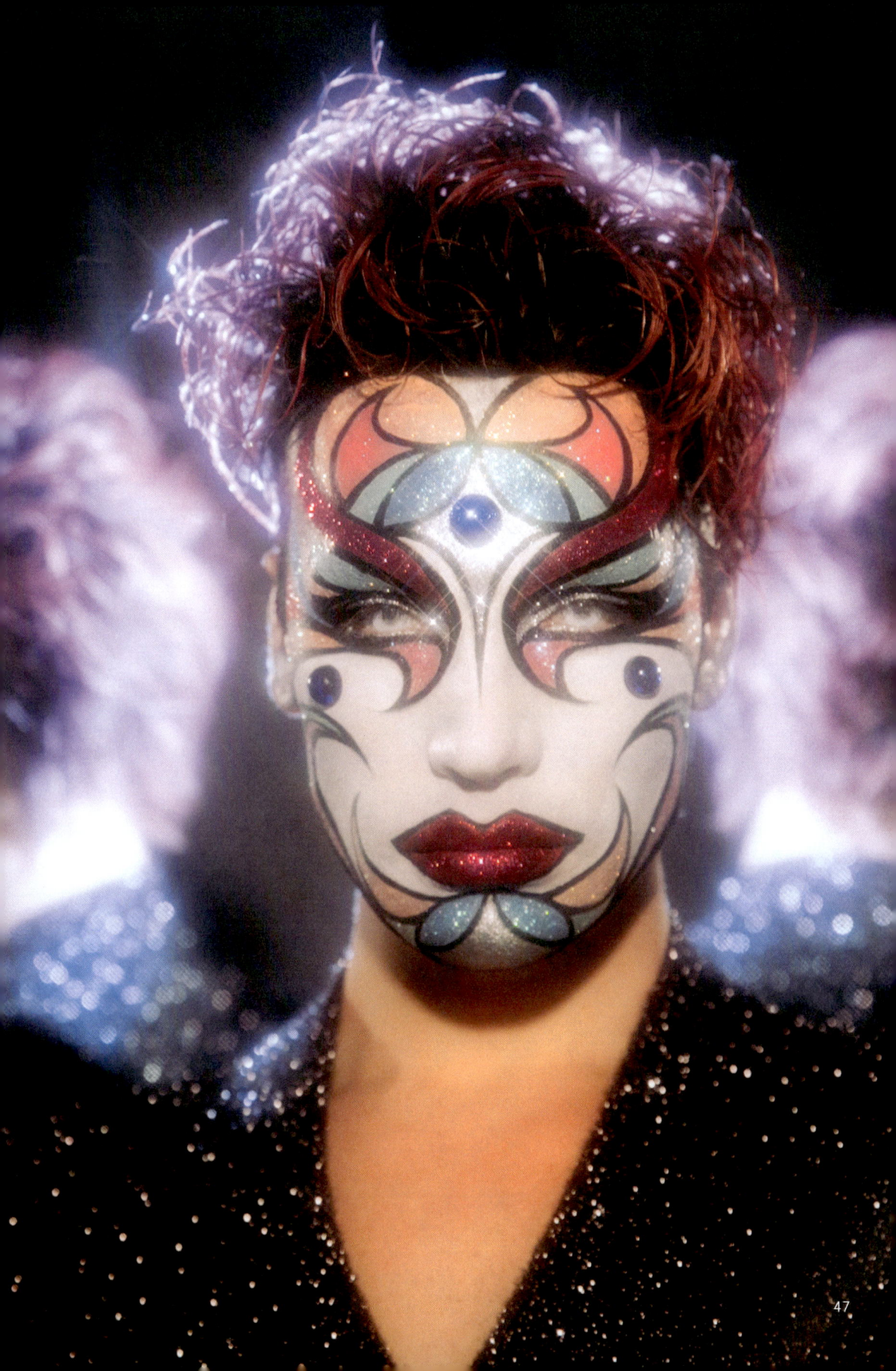

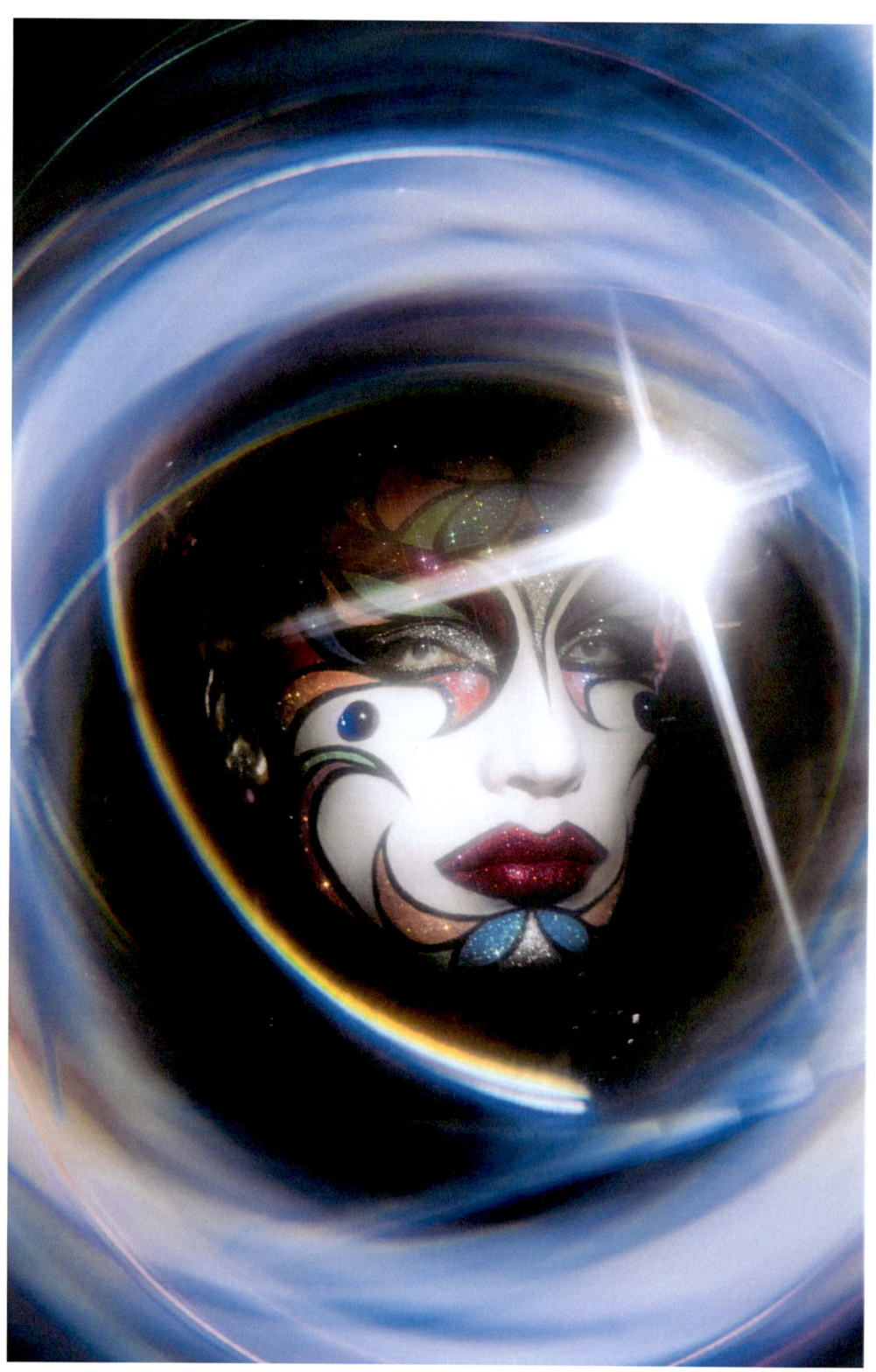

"Yeah, the MTV VMAs [Video Music Awards] happened, and that was wild." He recalls, "I guess you have this perspective based off of being the viewer—the fan, the spectator—and then you're behind the scenes. It's just very surreal, all these people walking around, doing their thing, working the stage."

At the awards show, Dahling helped craft Roan's ethereal Joan of Arc-inspired look, blending shades of gold, burgundy, and amber to complement her look. "She wanted to look like a medieval porcelain doll […] very hallowed, dreamy, and ethereal."

Standing backstage, Dahling says he couldn't help but think of the iconic VMA moments through the years that have shaped gay culture—and how he now had a hand in shaping another legendary VMA performance.

"I just thought of the Gaga VMA days, and how important those were to us when we were in high school. I still watch it, like all the time," he reflects.

2024 wasn't all glitter and spotlights, though. As Dahling puts it, "I've been saying that this is the best and worst year of my life. So much of the success came at a time when I was not doing super well." But even in those moments, the show must go on. "I understood these are once-in-a-lifetime opportunities to work with somebody like this. And not just, you know, the popularity that she has, [or even] how talented and amazing she is, but just aesthetically."

She's all I've ever wanted to do makeup on. She is that person. There were so many reasons why I was like, 'Okay, I cannot fuck this up. I cannot let my mental state get the best of me.'"

One of the most pivotal moments this year, both for Dahling and Roan, was Roan's debut on *Saturday Night Live*. "We weren't sure if it was going to happen or not, but at the last minute they decided to go for it. Both days were, like, 14-hour days. It was really intense," he recounts.

"But nobody knew that Kamala was coming, so we were all gagged." He explained how they suddenly cleared the hallway, and it was immediately flooded with Secret Service while Harris waited to go on for her skit. "So, that was kind of crazy."

Beyond sold out festivals and live television performances, Dahling finds inspiration in the vibrant and theatrical world of On Top, a party series put on by the legendary Suzanne Bartsch in NYC. "She's just such an important gay icon. She invented this whole [club kid] space. To work for her, do her makeup, and be a part of her life in general is so special."

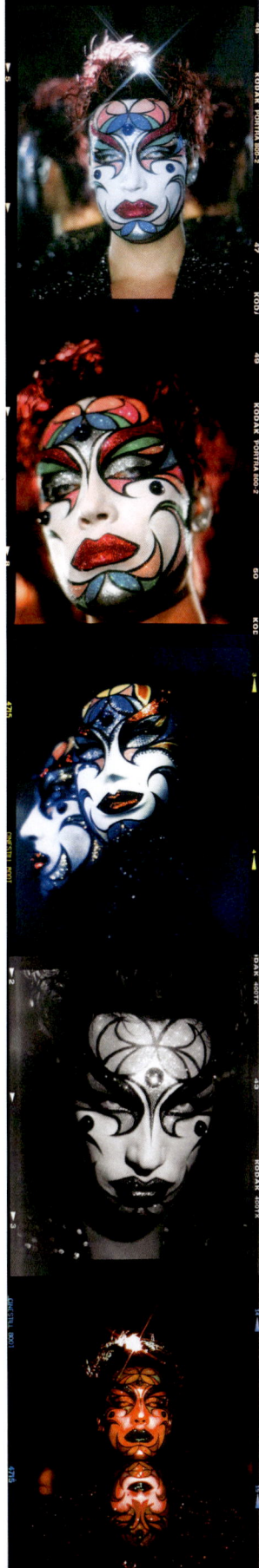

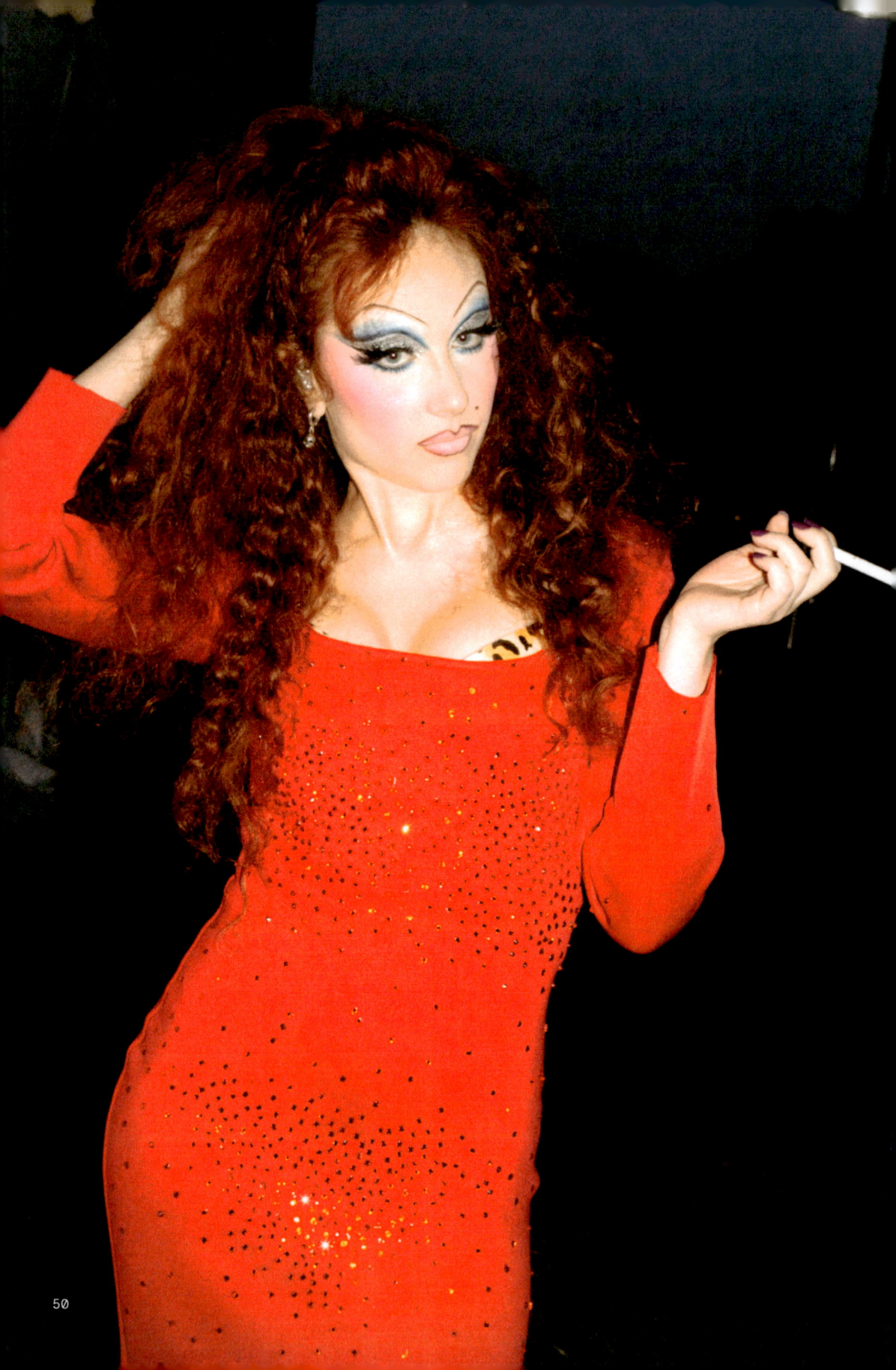

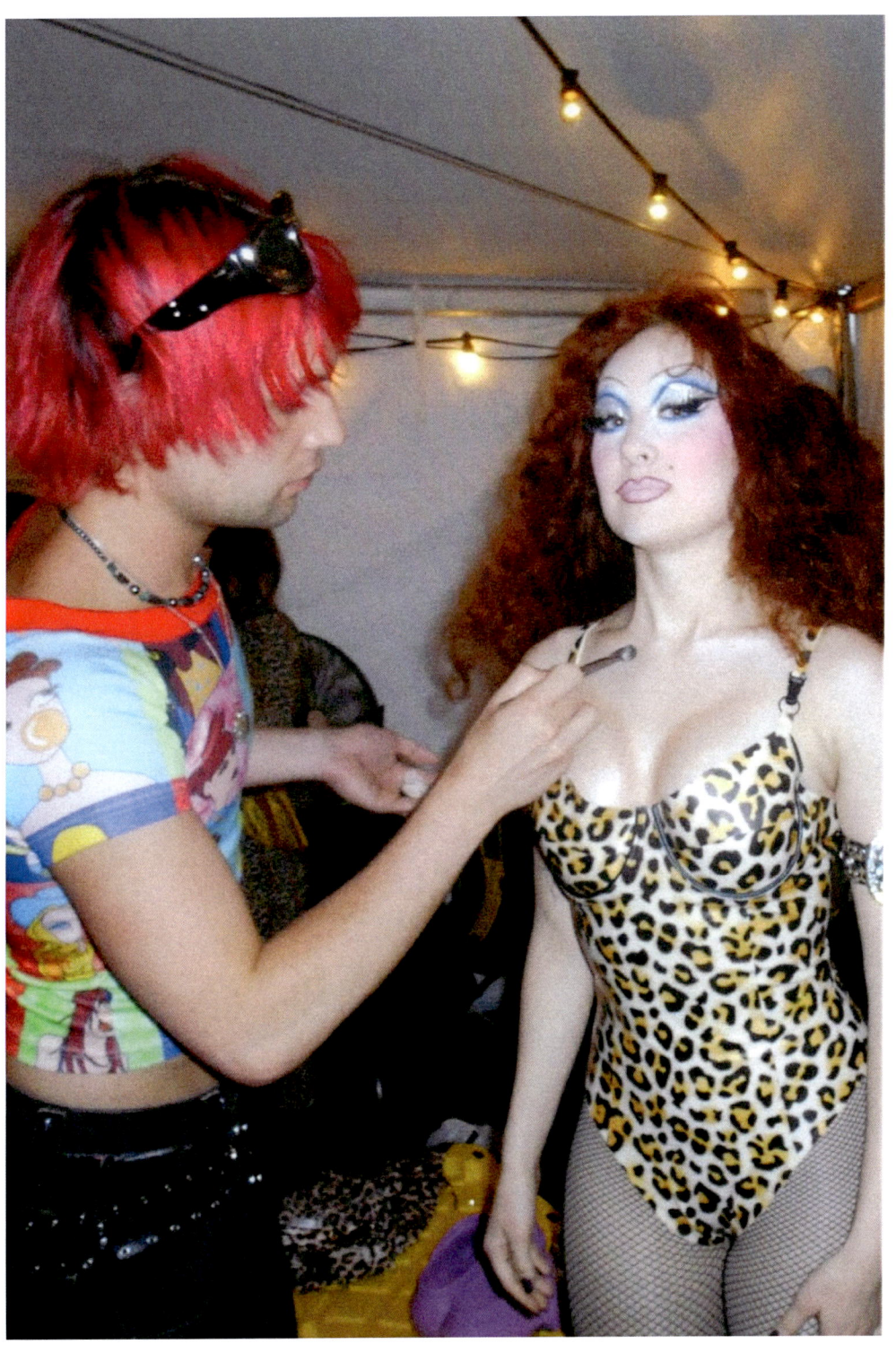

Above: Andrew Dahling paints Chappell Roan, photo courtesy of Andrew Dahling
Left: Chappell Roan as "Divine" at the Kentuckiana Pride Festival, photo courtesy of Chappell Roan

THE MOST INTENSE FEELING I HAVE IS
GRATITUDE

"All I wanted was to be a club kid in New York. And [On Top] really inspires my personal style too, as a makeup artist. It's another thing in my life that [just makes me] feel so lucky. I can't believe I actually get to be a part of this."

But as Dahling reflects on his journey from Boone County to the city, he hasn't forgotten his small-town roots. "There's this thing with New Yorkers—they kind of all understand and know that people that come here from small towns are always the ones that make it."

He went on, describing what it's like when you first get to the big city, "You have these big dreams, and you're working towards it, but you don't really know what it's going to be like when you actually get there. And you don't know for sure if you're going to get there. But then you do."

"Genuinely, the most intense feeling I have is gratitude. I just feel extremely lucky, like I just won the lottery or something. There's something about coming from such a small town and experiencing that for majority of your life, and then coming and creating a whole new life. If anything, it allows me to appreciate it more."

There's still so much for Dahling to do, though, and when asked about how his small-town definition of success has changed, he said, "I think for me, success is sort of like exploring the other sides of my creativity. It's so cliché to say this, but when you finally get somewhere that you feel like is pretty notable, and the dust settles, there's still all of these other things that you want to do."

"I want to get more into making my own clothes, and just taking the Andrew Dahling world—brand—into the next era. I'll never give [makeup] up completely, but things have been put into perspective with the state of the world. Nothing seems real. Everything's changing so fast. And I'm just at a point where I want to do everything I can possibly do before I die or I get old."

Dahling's humility and gratitude shine through every step of his story: "I'm so, so grateful that you all even care to do an interview with me. It's honestly such a huge honor." Whether it's working at the MAC store in Northern Kentucky, painting Chappell Roan's face for international audiences, or becoming a fixture of the club kid scene in New York City, his story is proof that persistence and creativity can open doors you never thought possible. From Boone County to Bartschland, his journey is far from over—and the Andrew Dahling world is only just beginning.

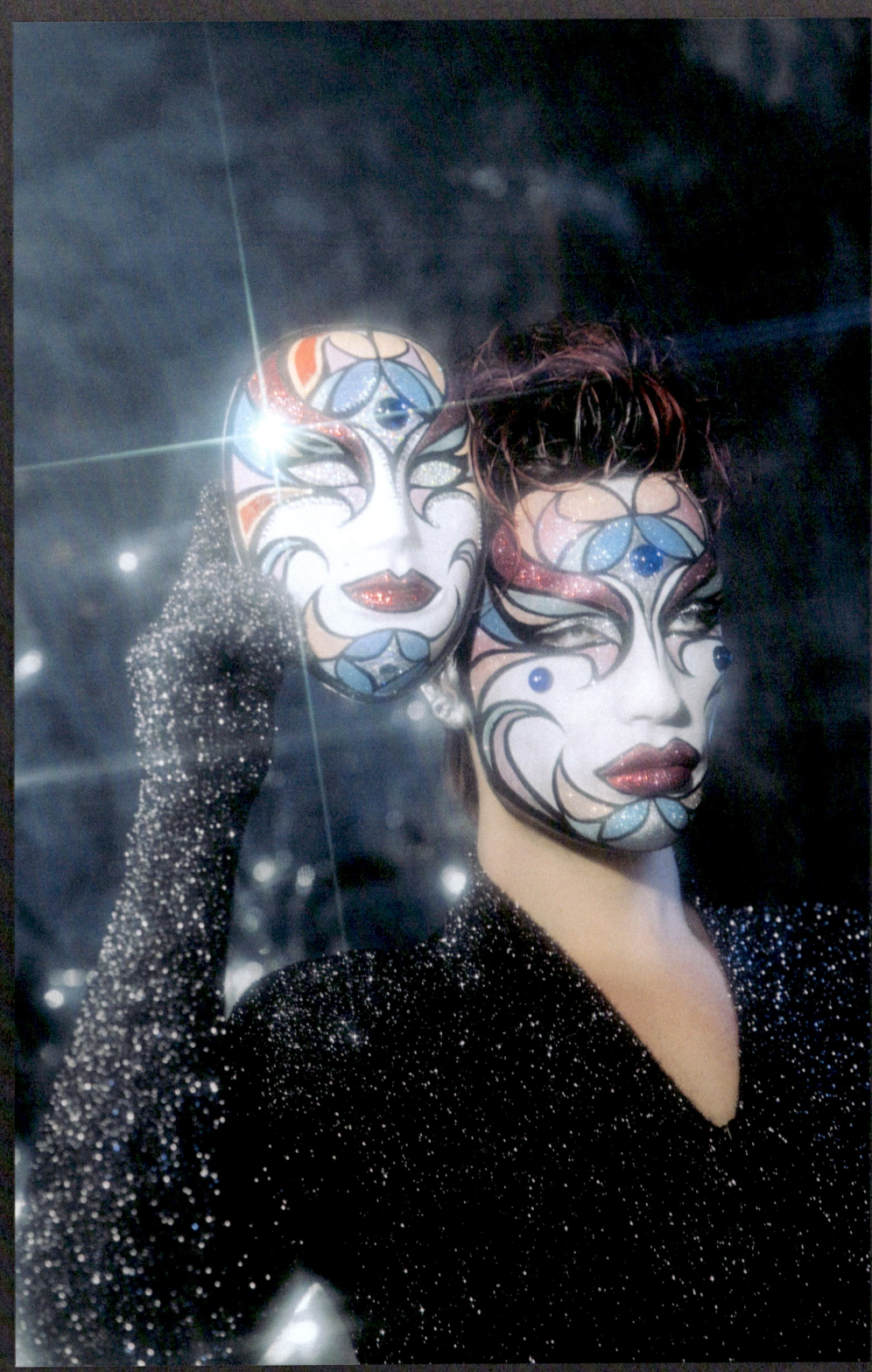

Performing Our Power

QUEER ADVOCACY IN THE BLUEGRASS STATE

Basel Touchan he/him @b_touchen

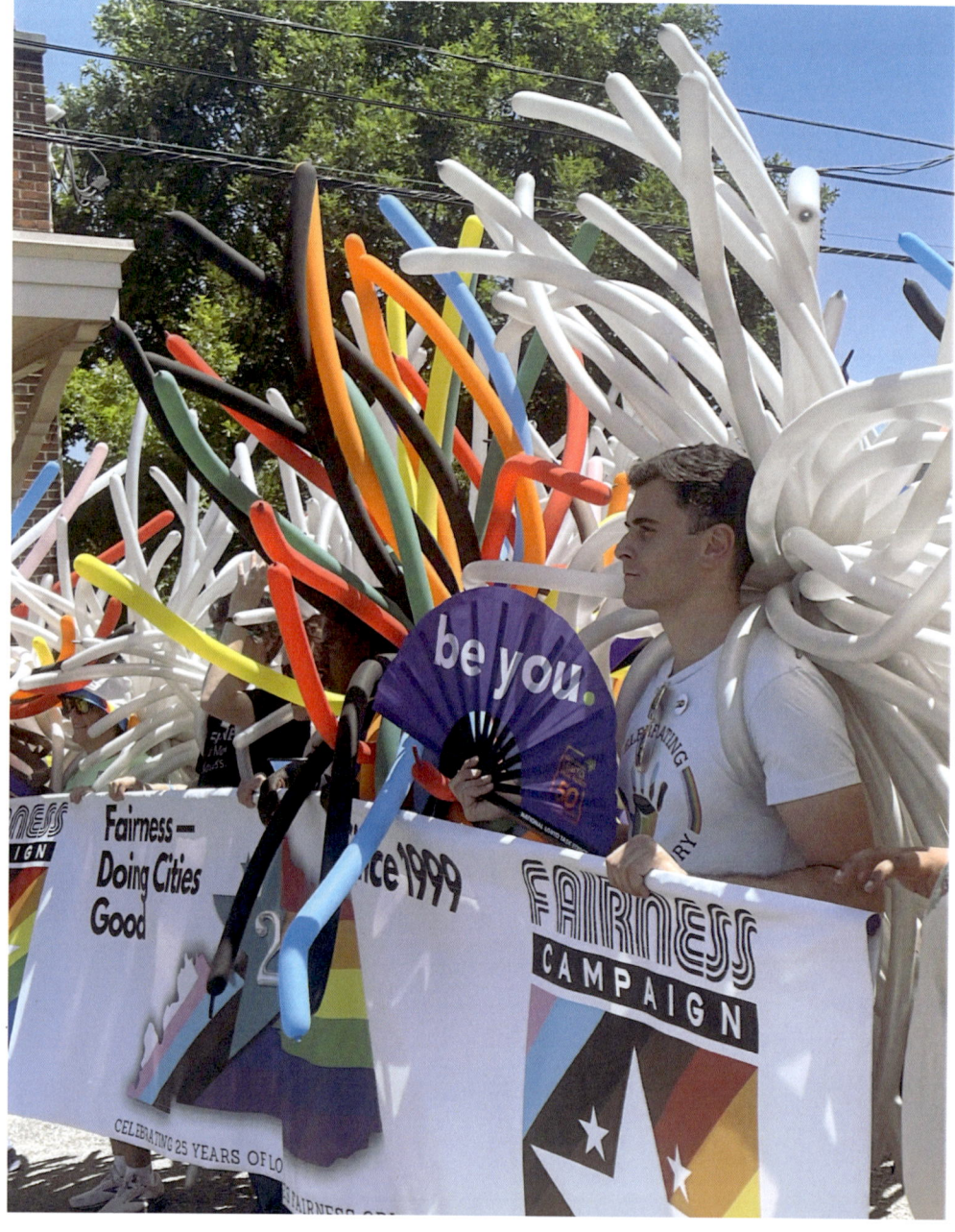

photo courtesy of Basel Touchan

If you've spent time in Lexington's Queer scene, you've probably heard the debate about where Pride should be held. For those outside the loop, let me get you up to speed.

In 2023, Lexington Pride moved to the Central Bank Convention Center instead of its former home at Robert F. Stephens Courthouse Plaza. Though both venues are only a brisk five-minute walk apart, it stirred quite a heated conversation. While some applauded the improved layout, the enhanced sense of safety, and the sweet relief of air-conditioning (who can forget that sweltering 86-degree festival in 2022?), others worried about costs for attendees, reduced revenue for nearby Queer and Queer-friendly businesses, and a loss of public visibility.

Whichever scenario you preferred likely depended on how you view the true purpose of Pride: is it a safe, joyful space for our own community and its allies, or is it a platform for advocacy and visibility in the broader Lexington and central Kentucky area?

There's value in both approaches to Pride. Take Louisville, for example, which hosts two Pride festivals—Kentuckiana Pride and Louisville Pride—where thousands fill the Big Four Lawn or flock to Bardstown Road. The city also has a huge parade, complete with Kentucky Fairness marching in signature balloon wings so iconic you'll see them in photos at SDF airport. Louisville's "show up big" philosophy runs deep. It's the city of Muhammad Ali, after all. Louisville was home to the first lesbian couple to sue for a legal marriage license in US history, as well as the first Lesbian Gay Liberation Front Kentucky chapter. More recently, Jefferson County Public Schools bussed students to Frankfort to protest SB150, despite ever-growing threats from the legislature.

The contrast between Louisville's and Lexington's approaches to Queer activism may come off stark—Lexington doesn't currently have a Pride march, for example. But, let's not forget that Fayette County was the first county in the state to pass a fairness ordinance, the first to elect an openly gay mayor, and the first to erect historical markers celebrating LGBTQ+ history and to paint rainbow crosswalks on public streets. Even in the days of Sweet Evening Breeze—a Black Queer icon long before Stonewall—the city found ways to celebrate its Queer leaders.

Some may attempt to draw broader conclusions here or even pit Kentucky's only two blue dots against each other. I prefer to leave that to the basketball court. In my opinion, neither city is "better" at Queer advocacy, but each of them contribute something unique by leaning into their own personality and culture to get things done.

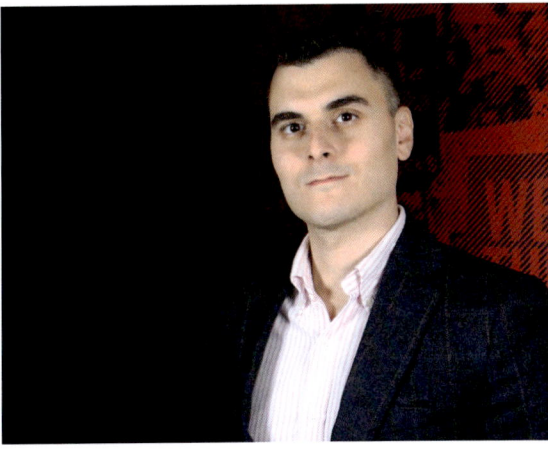

The question of how boldly or quietly we push for our rights has shaped Queer activism for generations. Queer activists have always balanced authenticity with relatability, navigating the need to center our vibrant rainbow of identities while also trying to gain traction in the monochromatic halls of power. This tension, this dance, has shaped LGBTQ+ movements from the 1950s to the present day. It even fractured the Mattachine Society, the first national gay and lesbian movement that ultimately launched the Gay Liberation Front in the wake of the Stonewall riots.

Think of gay activists like Frank Kameny, who initially insisted men wear suits and women wear dresses in 1960s protests because he believed it made the protests more palatable and impactful. Years later, he stormed the American Psychiatric Association's meetings to demand the removal of homosexuality as

photo courtesy of ACLU of Kentucky

We in Kentucky have one ace up our sleeve—we hate bullies and value authenticity above almost anything else.

a mental disorder from the DSM. Again and again, we see that both raucous protest and strategic compromise are essential to progress.

Mastering different approaches is key, especially in a red state as the political and societal winds continue to shift against our mere existence. However, I do not share the doom and gloom others may feel.

We in Kentucky have one ace up our sleeve— we hate bullies and value authenticity above almost anything else. Sure, Appalachia suffers from endless stereotypes, but as a Middle Easterner who's called Lexington my good ol' Kentucky home for almost a decade, I've encountered some of the warmest, most accepting folks in the hills and hollers. They might judge you, but they'll judge you on three things primarily: your work ethic, your kindness to neighbors, and whether you're true to yourself.

In my experience, the most impactful way to perform political advocacy in Kentucky is to not perform… at all. To shift hearts and minds, you simply need to show up visibly, vulnerably, and honestly. People around here can sniff out inauthenticity in a heartbeat.

Governor Andy Beshear is a prime example of someone who shows up without performing. He is steadfast in his support for activists, standing unapologetically with them at events and press conferences. He has also vetoed hateful legislation like SB150, fully aware the veto is only symbolic with a Republican supermajority and would be weaponized against him.

Despite all that, the majority of Kentuckians respected Beshear's allyship—even if they didn't agree with his views—because it felt genuine and true to his character. Imperfect as he may be (what politician isn't?), his sincerity resonates in a state that prizes honesty over spectacle.

Simply put, there isn't one "right way" to do Queer advocacy. We need the fiery passion that marches through the streets, and we also need the quiet, strategic deal-making that slips past the gates. Sometimes we'll be loud, sometimes we'll be pragmatic, but we'll always be working toward a Kentucky in which we can live, love, and celebrate our truths.

We all have a role to play this year. Go attend a local rally or city council meeting, volunteer for a grassroots campaign, or donate to organizations doing the on-the-ground work. Better yet, run for office yourself. And don't forget, how we show up matters as much as showing up at all.

Dr. Basel Touchan is the affiliate equity officer on the board of the ACLU of Kentucky, a board member of the New Americans Initiative, and vice chair of the Mayor's International Affairs Advisory Commission in Lexington, Ky.

nymph(o)

A queer, sex-positive magazine

nymphomagazine.info@gmail.com
nymphomagzine.com
@nympho.magazine

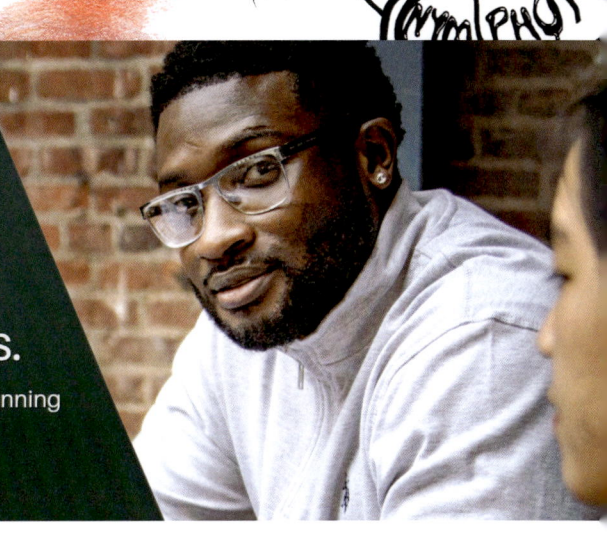

GRIMES
AND ASSOCIATES, LLC

We love working with **Dreamers**, even if you use a different word for dreams.

Bookkeeping | Financial Consulting | Payroll | Tax Planning

grimesandassociatesllc.com

✨ Business support that meets you where you are!

Inclusive and training-focused business support

Website Design | Branding Design
Graphic Design | Marketing Support

Alight Agency is Queer, Appalachian, and Woman Owned, ready to help you run your business with confidence and joy. ✨

AlightAgency.com | @AlightAgency | (859) 351-3542

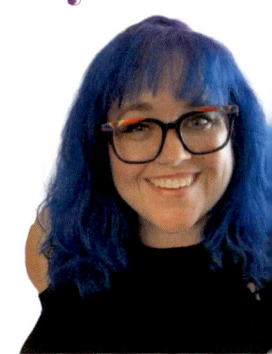

Your local hub for LGBTQIA support and community resources

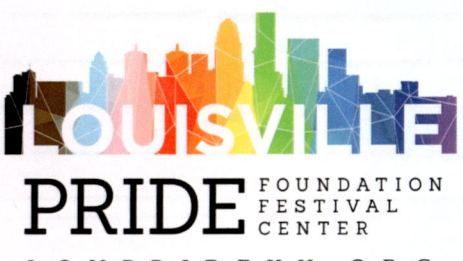

LOUISVILLE
PRIDE FOUNDATION FESTIVAL CENTER
LOUPRIDEKY.ORG

MEETING SPACES
SOCIAL EVENTS
LEARNING PROGRAMS
HARM REDUCTION KITS
AND MUCH MORE!

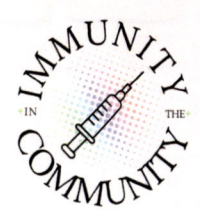

VACCINE CLINICS
COMING SOON

1244 S. Third Street Louisville, KY 40203 | 502-498-4298 | info@LouPrideKY.org

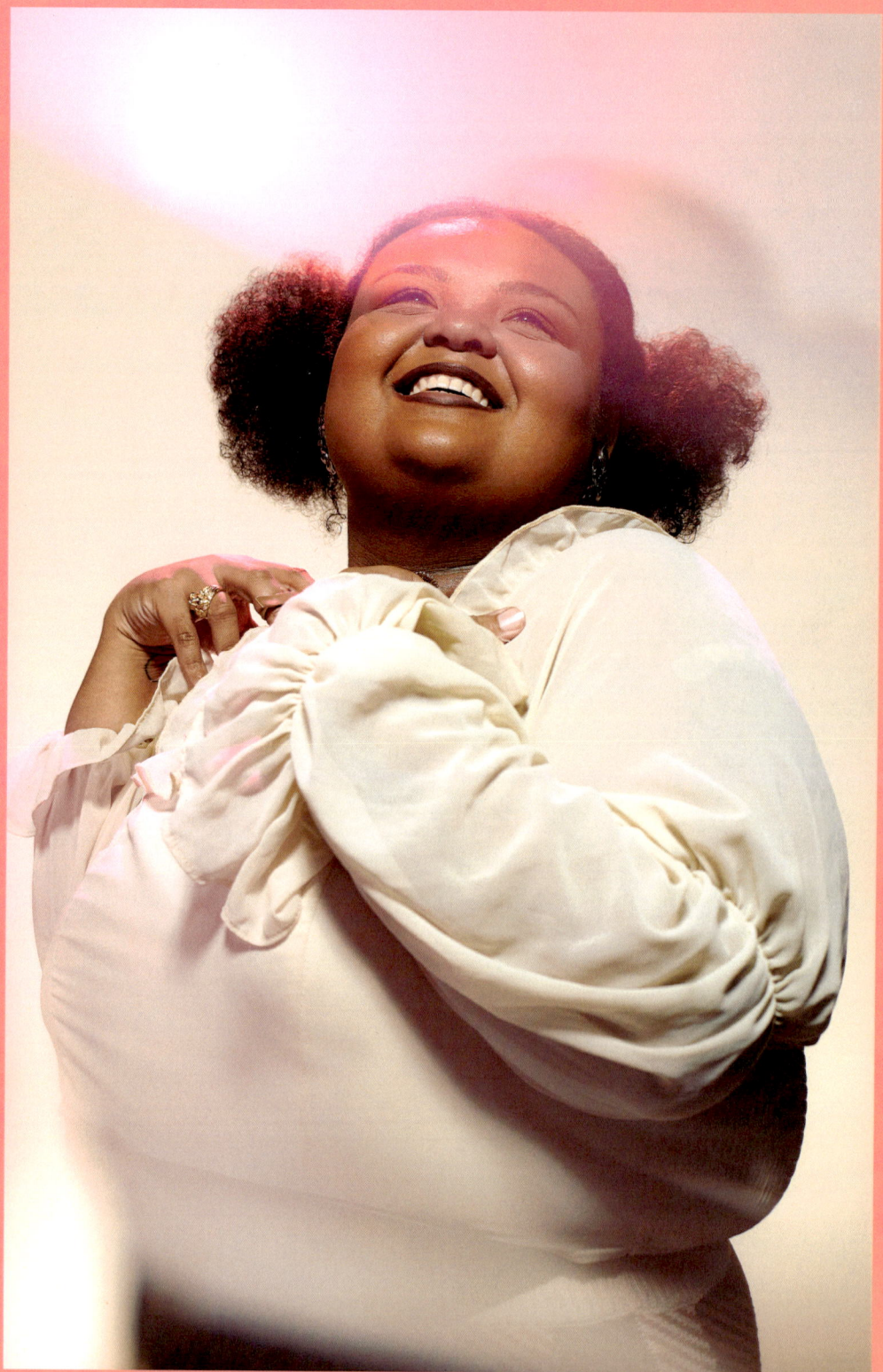

Images by Ryan Grant he/him @ryngrant

NEEDING NO MEETING PLACE

Sirene Martin she/her @sirenewata

Performance as an embodied modality of living has always been a central theme in my life. When I Googled the definition of "performance," I was intrigued by the way the sentence begins: "an act of...". These three words, I believe, capture the essence of performance. Initially, I thought performance had to involve some illusory or fictitious component, but I soon realized that the practice of performance extends beyond stage presentations. If I base my understanding of performance on "an act of...," I can include societal roles such as parenting, mentoring, and teaching—all of which, to some extent, are forms of performance. I embody performance through my career, my artistic practice, my relationships, and more. However, on the flip side, we live in a society that pressures individuals to conform to a dominant narrative of performance, a narrative rooted in the United States' foundations of white supremacy, anti-Blackness, and Christian extremism. As a result, roles like gender and race are often tainted by misogyny, anti-Black bias, and Christian dogma.

From an early age, I learned the importance of performance, primarily through a raced lens in which, as a Black person, I must always be keenly aware of white people. I must be aware of the way I talk, how they talk to me, and what I share with them. Every Black child is taught the language of the oppressing class as a form of protection. As I grew older and began to notice things about myself, I became acutely aware that I was different from my family and peers at school. Although it was unintelligible to me at the time, the person I am now can clearly see what set me apart, and that is my Queer identity. It is important for me to define my understanding of Queerness as it relates to me. My existence is Queer because it lives outside the limits of white cis-heteronormativity. To me, Blackness is inherently Queer in this way. At this time, I will not situate myself at an intersection where sexuality, gender, and race meet—because in my life, they have never been separate and need no meeting place.

As a trans woman, performance has been crucial for my sense of self and my mental well-being. It has also been both a tool for safety and a source of heartache. I often reflect on the early stages of my transition, particularly the times when I was frequently misgendered. I think about how much I had to focus on my appearance and dress, as it felt like a form of policing. Those mornings often felt like experiments. I spent a lot of time thinking about what skirt, shapewear, jewelry would make me small enough to digest for the male gaze. Before medically transitioning, I felt burdened by my body. Now, years removed from that time, all I can remember is feeling scared, stressed, and utterly uneasy in my body.

A vital aspect of performance is the audience. What do they think? How do they perceive you, and what are their takeaways? These thoughts are exhausting to carry every day. My early morning thoughts were consumed with the desire to pass. I wanted to create a canyon of separation between the person and gender that had been imposed upon me and the person and soul I've always known myself to be. This desire to widen that divide led me down very toxic paths of femininity, often rooted in patriarchy and anti-Blackness. I sought to make myself smaller, to speak softer, to wear clothing and accessories that were considered hyper-feminine. if I'm honest with myself, I sought validation from the male gaze.

When I think about my womanhood, I think about my mother. As a child, whenever I was asked what I wanted to be when I grew up, my immediate thought was always my mother. This made me feel a bit odd, as no one else seemed to want to be like their parents. I grew up mesmerized by her—she was my first friend and role model. I revered her power and the way she commanded respect. I admired how she could captivate a room and an audience. She was humorous and quite the songstress of her time and community. My desire to be close to her, and to the women in my family, has grounded the performance I call life. There were moments in my childhood when it felt as though I was living behind a double mirror: I could see out, but others couldn't see me. I remember being organized in school or church by "boys go here" and "girls go there," and

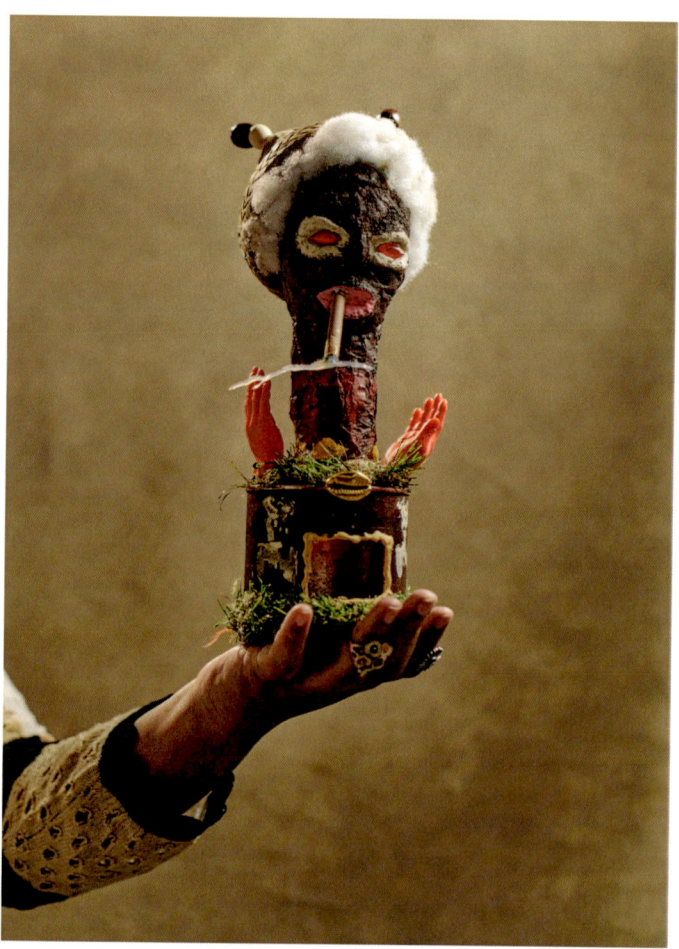

Martin displays her sculpture that is symbolic of her of journey through the self. The figure is comprised of found objects which reflect her understandings of identity formation. A gathering of unlikely and likely items to create a new thing.

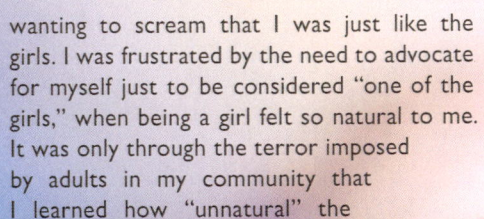

wanting to scream that I was just like the girls. I was frustrated by the need to advocate for myself just to be considered "one of the girls," when being a girl felt so natural to me. It was only through the terror imposed by adults in my community that I learned how "unnatural" the world saw me.

I feel terribly confused writing this. Thinking of performance has sparked an interest and analysis of my personhood through the lens of time and unlearning. I am trying to make sense of a journey that seems to have no clear rhyme or reason, and in this attempt, I feel as though I am over-intellectualizing myself. All I've ever wanted is to exist in the simple, quiet, and grounded space of being. I envy those who seemingly erupt into this life without the burden of self-actualization.

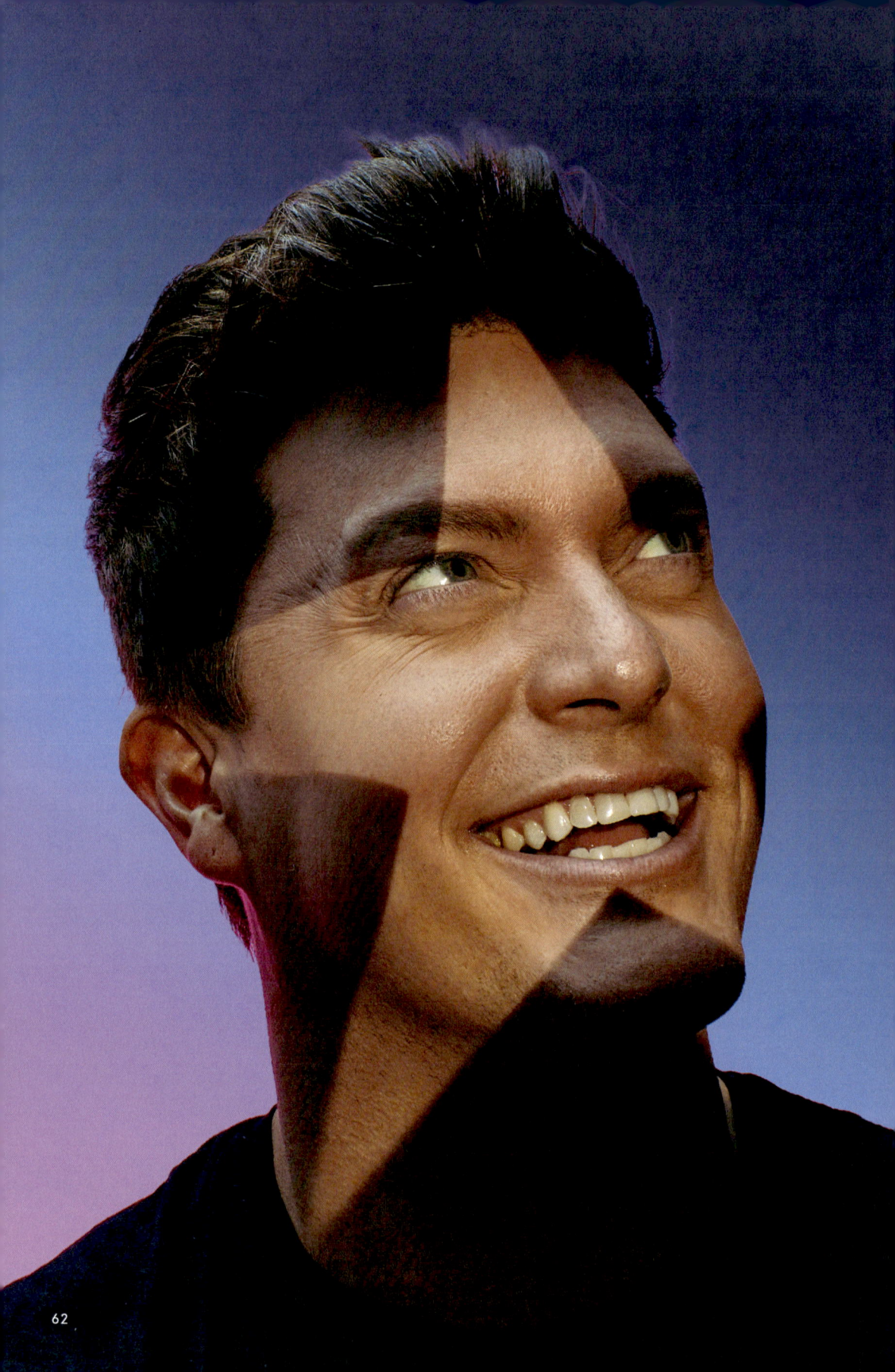

ZACK WICKHAM'S LOVE LETTER TO LOUISVILLE

FROM GROWING UP IN THE PROGRESSIVE HEART OF KENTUCKY TO SHINING A LIGHT ON LGBTQ+ STORIES IN BRAVO'S THE VALLEY

Missy Spears she/they @missy.spears

As Zack Wickham, star of Bravo's hit show *The Valley*, glides into a photography studio located on Whiskey Row in Downtown Louisville, he's holding his clothes in one hand, offering hugs with the other, and rattling off his favorite facts about his favorite city to his boyfriend, Benji.

"Did you know Louisville produces more disco balls than anywhere else in the world? Or that Louisville has the best tap water in the country?"

Images by Ryan Grant he/him @ryngrant

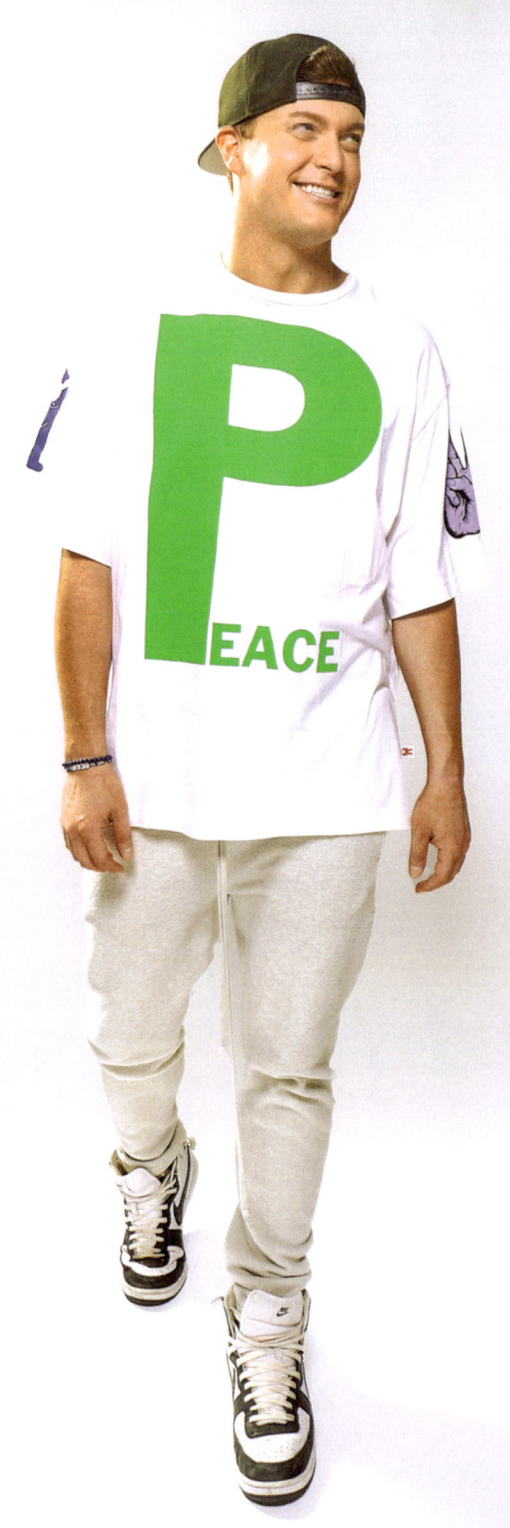

For those of you not in the Bravo universe, I'm happy to be your tour guide. Wickham stars in *The Valley*, a breakout hit reality show that first aired in 2024 as a spinoff to *Vanderpump Rules*, aka VPR. VPR was launched in 2013 as a sneak peek into the antics of service industry staff (raise your hand if you've ever worked at a restaurant and fucked a coworker) and quickly became one of the network's top shows. While the show lacked any real diversity, we lived for our bisexual sandwich shop queen Ariana Maddix and enjoyed every second of one Tom in a dress crying over another Tom in a dress, who is clearly trying to take a shit in private.

But as it happens in life, friend groups shift. People break up, couple up, move to the suburbs, and spit out kids. *The Valley* was launched off of this change, bringing back former VPR stars Jax Taylor and Kentucky native, Brittany Cartwright, along with their real-life friend group, which of course includes Cartwright's best friend of fifteen years, Zack Wickham.

"I did *Vanderpump Rules* for years and years where I was the new person," Cartwright said. "And I came to a new show where I didn't know anybody, and luckily they were all great to me, but it can be very intimidating. So to start off with *The Valley*, I knew like 1000% that Zack had to be on the show with me. He has been one of my best friends for over 15 years now. And it wouldn't be my real life or our friend group's real life if he wasn't a huge part of that."

Unlike most Hollywood stars, Wickham didn't leave for Los Angeles until he was older. "I had a full adult life before moving to LA at 29, which feels late to make such a big leap," he says.

In Louisville, Wickham was deeply entrenched in the LGBTQ+ community: interning for Fairness Campaign Executive Director Chris Hartman, obtaining his master's at Bellarmine University, and enjoying the world-class drag production that beloved LGBTQ+ club, The Connection (rest in peace), brought to the city.

"There was so much stuff like that that I take pride in. I kind of grew up on the best of the best of the LGBT community" he says. "Every time I come back, I get to relive all those memories in a city that's changed in all the right ways but stayed true to itself where it matters."

Moving from Louisville to LA created quite the culture shock for the Trinity High graduate and his start was a little rocky.

"My first year in LA, I spent $3,000 on parking tickets and towing fees. It's such a typical 'I-just-moved-to-LA' story,'" Wickham laughs. "Luckily I did have Brittany, who I knew before she was on Vanderpump Rules. Then when I started hanging out with her, that group became my friend group, and I luckily was integrated very fast into that, so that I didn't have to worry about finding friends."

But, as many of us can relate, the pandemic changed a lot of that. During this time,

EVERY TIME I COME BACK, I GET TO RELIVE ALL THOSE MEMORIES IN A CITY THAT'S CHANGED IN ALL THE RIGHT WAYS BUT STAYED TRUE TO ITSELF WHERE IT MATTERS.

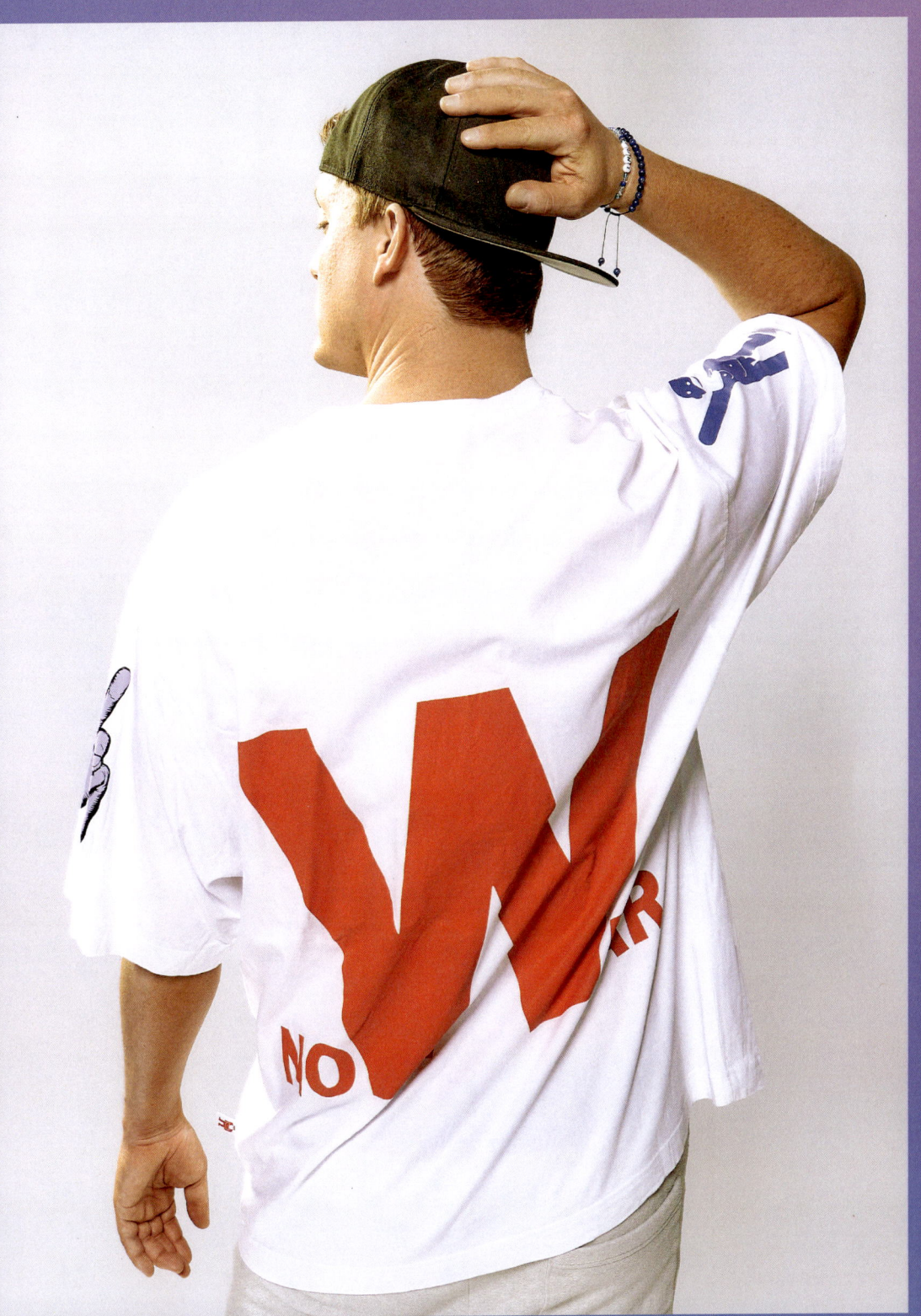

THE SHOW MUST GO ON 67

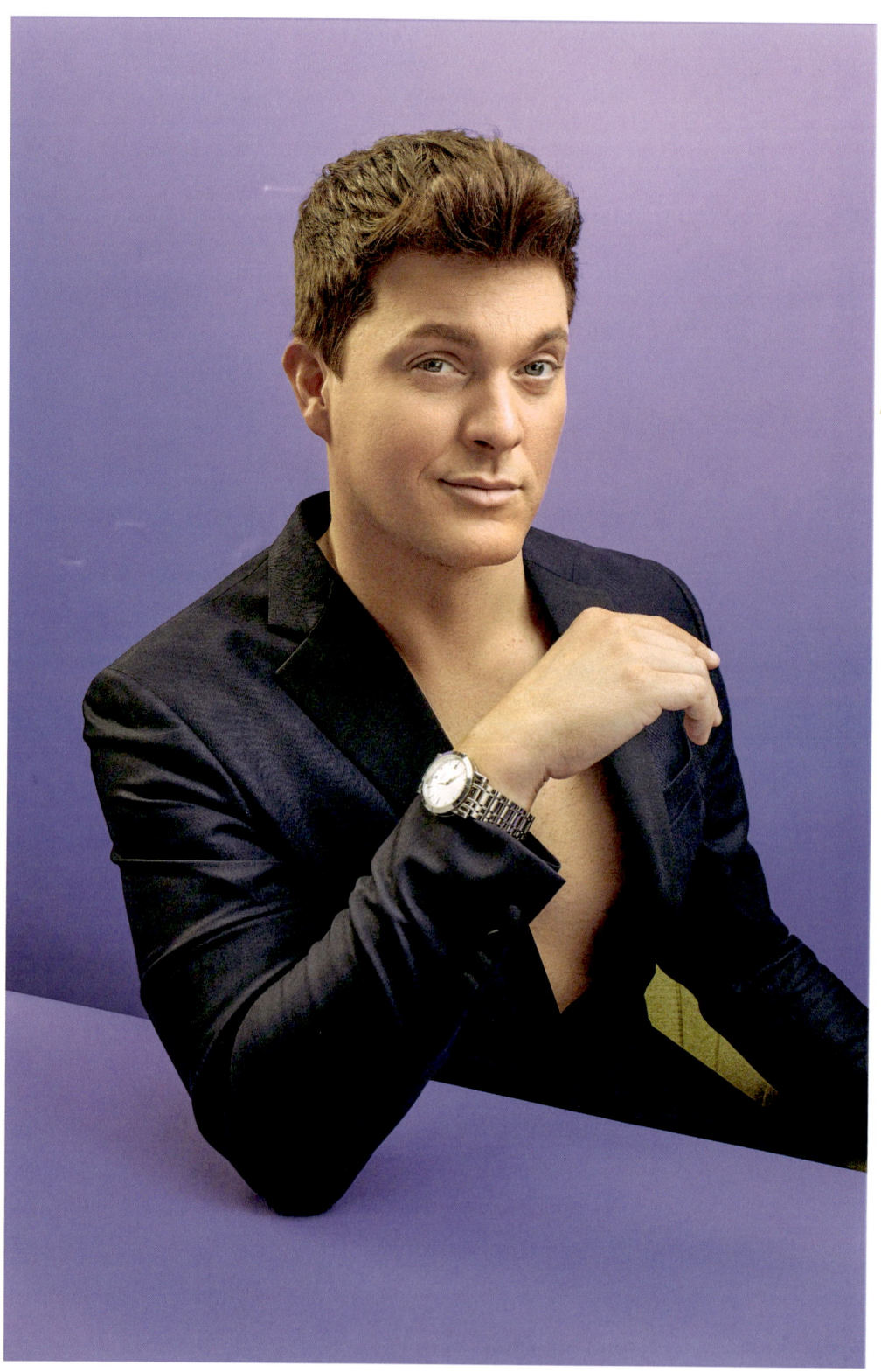

Wickham was separated from Cartwright and their shared friend group, many of them protecting new and immunocompromised family members. This provided an opportunity for him to build a foundation of LGBTQ+ friends and support that he was missing in LA.

"Even on *The Valley*," Wickham says, "it's all about families and heteronormativity. And that's great. You can have friends and they can understand to a degree of stuff, but they'll never know what you as a gay man goes through or as a Queer person goes through and so it's really nice to have that to fall back on. And I think when my straight friends were busy with a lot of stuff I really realized how important having that community is because I had it in Louisville. And when I moved it was harder to find."

For season two of *The Valley*, Wickham is excited to share more of his life. During season two, cameras will now be following Wickham on his own storylines, showing glimpses of his happy relationship with boyfriend Benji, while also offering a peek into the life of somebody not at the same financial level as their friends.

"Being that I'm the poorest on the cast, you get to really see my life," he says with a laugh "And I think it's a view that you don't get with some of the other people because I'm struggling still."

He and his boyfriend won't be the only healthy, happy LGBTQ+ couple on the show—his close friend Jasmine Goode, recently engaged to Melissa Marie, will also be more heavily shown in season two.

Goode says, there haven't really been many reality shows that showcase the lives of Queer people and are excited to put Queer love front and center.

"So to be on a platform where they're allowing that, and they show our lives authentically, it's beautiful," she says "And I'm very thankful and I'm glad to do it with one of my best friends. Me and Zack have been friends for years, we used to live together. So now that we, you know, we used to live together, now we're on a show together, it's just wild. I love it."

Wickham said he is counting down the days to the premiere of season two of *The Valley* which premiers in April on Bravo and will be streaming the next day on Peacock.

"Well, I'll just say that I feel like every other or every third episode is almost like a finale. That's how crazy it is. There's always a cliffhanger, and every episode will probably have a cliffhanger, and every third episode will be, like, finale-level drama, because we are that intense right now. We've just gone through it."

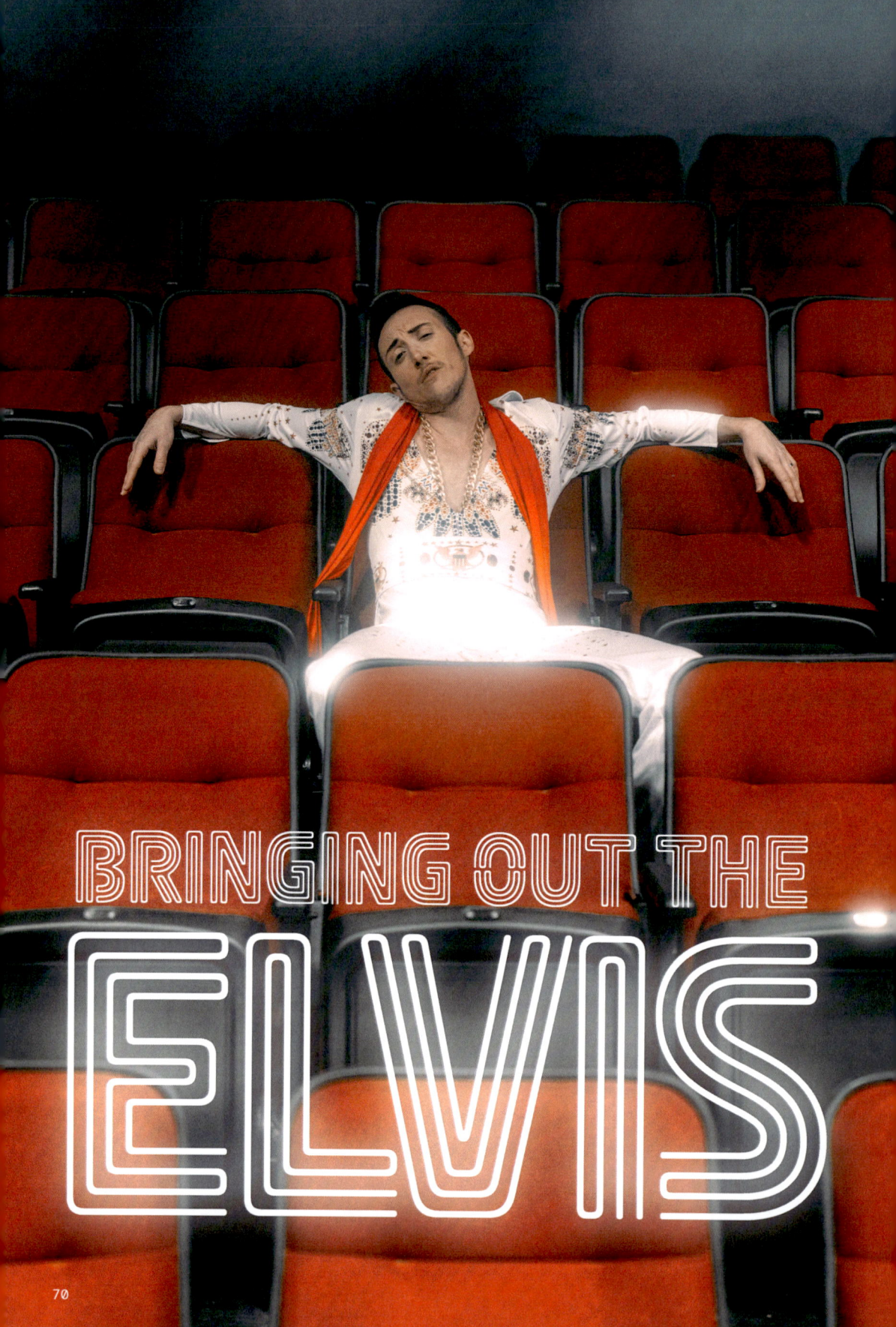

A RETROSPECTIVE ON THE BIRTH OF A DRAG KING
Vic Leon he/they @thevicleon

I stood on a rickety stage in front of my entire school with my head cast down. It was the middle school talent show, and I was about to lip sync You're Bringing Out the Elvis in Me by Faith Hill. I wore a pair of french braids and jean capris, a tank top, a tattoo choker, and Baby-Phats on my feet.

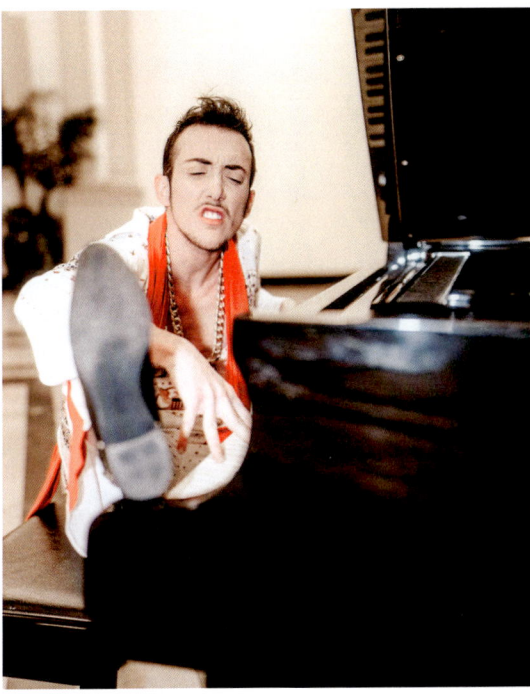

I took my starting position on stage and waited for the music. The country singer's voice blasted through the speakers inside the gym. I rocked with the beat. Swinging my hips with such gusto that I believed in that moment I was *the* Elvis Presley. The last twang of the harmonica rang out through the speakers as I stuck my last pose, anticipating a roar of applause.

But it never came.

As I finally met the audience's silent, bewildered stares, embarrassment washed over me. The ridicule that followed weeks after cemented my desire to fade into the background.

Now socially scarred, I settled on basketball to carry me through the rest of middle school. But my performance anxiety was too much, even on the court. By the time I was a sophomore, I ditched my high-tops for character shoes, finding the stage was a safer space to play with a script to guide me. In theater, I found true friends and also discovered I was gay. Though primarily closeted, the confidence to embrace myself began to grow, discovering there was a world that would accept me.

What's more, I couldn't deny that I loved to act and I wanted to do it for life. After five years as a museum actor and doing community theatre in Louisville, I realized that if I wanted to continue to grow as an actor and do it professionally, I needed formal training. I had a Bachelor of Arts in Theater from Bellarmine University but I knew I needed to go to the next level. I took a Greyhound to Chicago to audition for the University Resident Theatre Association, intent on landing a Masters of Fine Arts program that would take me as a student. I caught the eye of two different schools, and after callbacks, I had an offer from the University of Houston's Professional Actor Training Program with a full ride. I packed my bags and left Louisville, hoping for a brighter future doing what I loved.

The training at UH was hard, fast, and grueling from day one, and I devoted all that I had for two years. While I was the out and proud lesbian of my ensemble of eight, the program took a toll on me, and by my second year I wasn't feeling as confident as I did when I arrived. Something was shifting within me. My work became muddy, introspective, and distracted. Grad school stripped us down to rebuild us as actors, but instead of strength, I felt confusion and gnawing depression.

Images by Scotty Milks   he/him   @milkmanphotography

When it came time to decide what I wanted to do after grad school, I felt like I needed to go back to Louisville and be with my then-girlfriend. I returned to civilian life, learning that same year what non-binary meant. I found solace on the Internet with others like me, discovering that there were other options for an identity that felt more like my own experience with gender. It was a painful but necessary metamorphosis. And like I'd always done when I was unsure of where to go, I looked to the stage to find myself.

I secured some work in the last *Christmas Carol* that Actors Theatre of Louisville would see onstage. Then the world shut down and we entered the COVID-19 pandemic. My girlfriend and I broke up, and I thought maybe moving to Los Angeles would fix me as I was picking up the pieces of my broken heart and trying to "make it" on my own. It didn't, and I went back to Louisville with my tail between my legs, unsure of what to do with myself once again. I felt stuck in auditioning — my in-between gender was not reading to casting directors. They didn't know where to put me. I didn't know where to put me.

I returned to drag as a creative outlet, drawn back to it after performing a few open stages at Play Louisville before grad school. There was something about it that made things less chaotic inside me. Being a drag king gave me permission to extend myself and become my own creative salvation, allowing myself to embody a bold, electrified version of Vic that traditional roles never did. The more I leaned in, the more I found myself offstage. And then one day, fresh out the shower drying my legs, it hit me like a bolt from the blue:

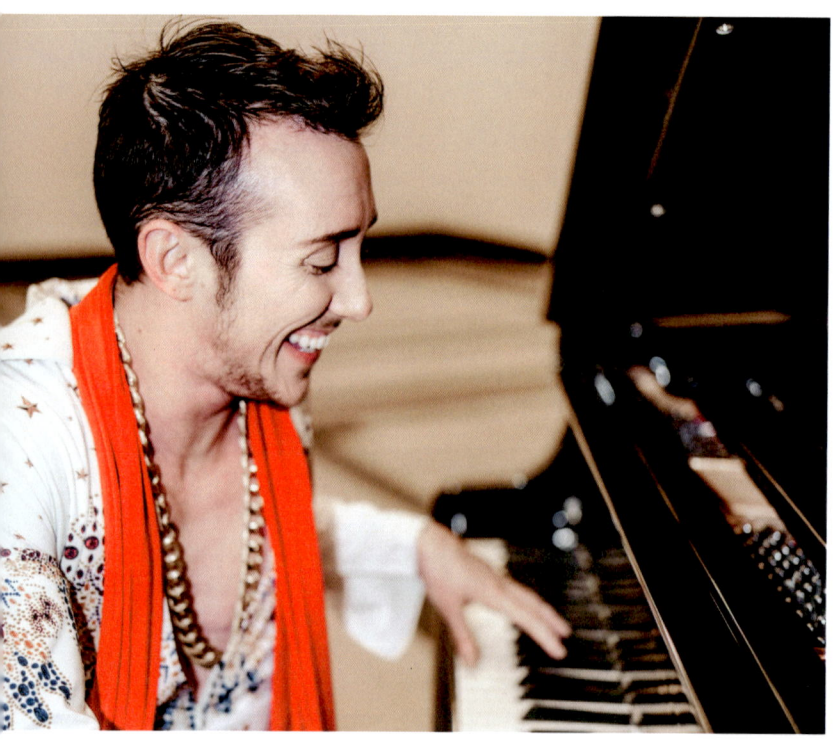

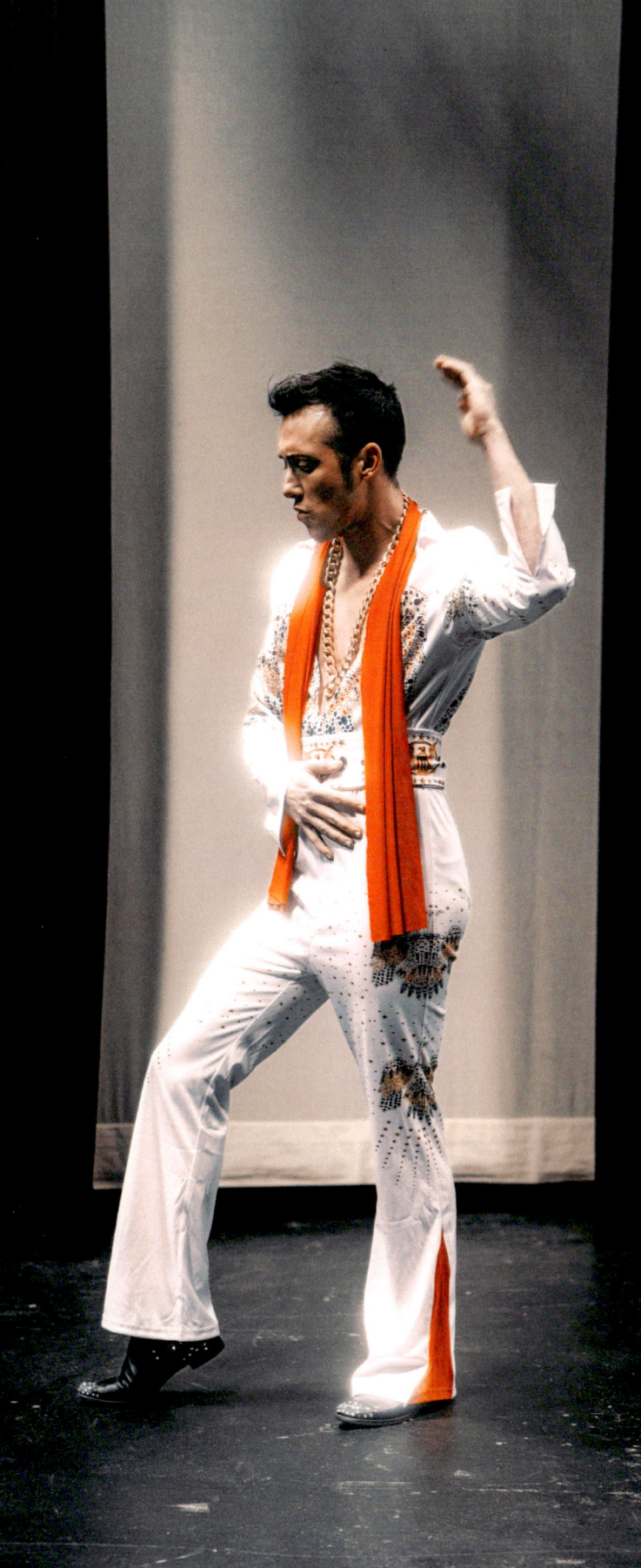

I'm transgender.

That realization illuminated my path, allowing me to take the steps to live authentically and confidently as a man. I stopped wearing dresses, bound my chest, started HRT, scheduled my top surgery, and worked at a phone store for insurance to cover the costs. As I made these subtle changes overtime, I began to notice how differently people treated me as a guy. It was a shift I felt deeply—no longer feeling out of place when I said "Thanks, man," or sat naturally in a chair. I felt how freeing it was to choose when and how we can evolve on our own terms. With self-awareness and unconditional love towards myself, my power began to grow. My spark came back brighter and stronger than ever.

Even in uncertain moments, I still channel the fearless kid on that rickety stage — so joyful and eager to share what it was that made him light up — without a care of what people might think of him. Like Elvis, all I ever wanted to do was share my joy with the world. And even if I didn't know it then, I was already making moves towards the person I was always meant to be.

ART IS A RIGHT NOT A PRIVILEGE

BECOME A PROUD SUPPORTER OF YOUR ARTS ECOSYSTEM AT FUNDFORTHEARTS.ORG TODAY.

www.ingramcontent.com/pod-product-compliance
Lightning Source LLC
Chambersburg PA
CBRC101145030426
42337CB00009B/75